The Immunological Basis of Surgical Science and Practice

The Immunological Basis of Surgical Science and Practice

Edited by

OLEG EREMIN

Regius Professor of Surgery
University of Aberdeen

and

HERB SEWELL

Professor of Immunology
University of Nottingham

Oxford New York Tokyo
OXFORD UNIVERSITY PRESS
1992

Oxford University Press, Walton Street, Oxford OX2 6DP

Oxford New York Toronto
Delhi Bombay Calcutta Madras Karachi
Petaling Jaya Singapore Hong Kong Tokyo
Nairobi Dar es Salaam Cape Town
Melbourne Auckland

and associated companies in
Berlin Ibadan

Oxford is a trade mark of Oxford University Press

Published in the United States
by Oxford University Press, New York

A catalogue record for this book is available from the British Library

Library of Congress Cataloging in Publication Data
(Data available)
ISBN 0-19-261933-0

Set by Colset Pte Ltd, Singapore
Printed and bound in Great Britain
by Bookcraft (Bath) Ltd
Midsomer Norton, Avon.

Preface

The aim of this book is to present an up-to-date, concise, and interesting account of immunology and its relevance to the clinical practice of surgery. Although there are many excellent textbooks on immunology, both large and small, few to date have been written predominantly for a surgical readership.

Immunology is a rapidly expanding biological science which has had a major impact on many aspects of medical practice, both diagnostic and therapeutic. Immunology is providing an insight into and offering an explanation for a number of disease processes in surgical practice (e.g., sepsis, trauma, cancer) and is responsible for the introduction of new and innovative therapy—cytokine and lymphokine-activated killer (LAK) cell infusions.

It is essential for the young surgical trainee to be informed of these important biological discoveries and to be aware of their possible impact on surgical practice. It is hoped, however, that the more established surgeon will also find this book of benefit in keeping abreast of developments in the 'new' biologies.

In Chapter 1, emphasis is placed on the cellular and molecular aspects of immunology, a knowledge of which has contributed to a greater understanding of normal immunity and its disturbance in various disease processes, particularly those with an underlying autoimmune basis. Subsequent chapters highlight contributions to those areas of medicine with direct relevance to surgical science and practice. These include transplantation (Chapter 2), cancer and host defences (Chapter 3), and the emerging appreciation of the immune response in trauma and severe sepsis (Chapters 4 and 5 respectively). The importance of nutrition on immune reactivity is discussed in Chapter 6, whilst modulation of the immune response by various treatment modalities employed to treat surgical patients is outlined in Chapter 7. Chapter 8 is a timely account of the relevance of autoimmunity to, and, in particular, the impact of AIDS on surgical practice. The final chapter aims to give an overview of the principles of some of the common techniques and assays used in modern molecular medicine-immunology, an area that many surgeons find difficulty in understanding, but a knowledge of which provides a framework in which to interpret the published data in the literature.

Equally, the Glossary is a valuable and readily available source of information on terms used in immunology. We have restricted the references and further reading to selected texts and articles. The interested reader can use them judiciously to acquire more information and/or detailed discussion relating to topics outlined or described in various chapters.

We are privileged to have a number of internationally renowned surgeons writing authoritatively on their area of expertise. Their valuable contributions to this book are much appreciated.

Aberdeen and Nottingham
January 1992

O.E.
H.F.S.

Contents

Contributors

J. Broom Department of Clinical Biochemistry, University of Aberdeen

W. Cheadle Department of Surgery, University of Louisville, USA

R. Dionigi Director of Surgery, University of Pavia-Várese, Italy

L. Dominioni Department of Surgery, University of Pavia-Várese, Italy

O. Eremin Regius Professor of Surgery, University of Aberdeen

H.C. Polk Jr. Ben A. Reid Sr. Professor and Chairman, Department of Surgery, University of Louisville, USA

H.F. Sewell Professor of Immunology, University of Nottingham

A. Thomson Reader in Pathology, University of Aberdeen

R.F.M. Wood Professor of Surgery, St. Bartholomew's Hospital, London

1
Basic immunology

H.F. Sewell

1.1 Introduction

The seeds of immunology took root in the fertile studies of infectious diseases by scientists in the eighteenth and nineteenth centuries. In the early twentieth century it grew as a sturdy sapling under the care of the immunochemists with continued input from microbiologists. By the mid-twentieth century immunology emerged as a fully grown science in its own right, with extensive branches in immunochemistry, cellular immunology, immunobiology, immunogenetics, and clinical immunology/immunopathology. In the latter part of the twentieth century, it continues to extend its branches and develop new blossoms; the biotechnologies of hybridomas, T cell and gene cloning, peptide synthesis, and the use of transgenic and chimeric animal models enrich and expand its development. An essential set of ingredients have continually contributed to the development of immunology. These are represented by *original concepts*, imaginative basic *experimental research*, astute *clinical observations*, and *technological* advances. The continued interactions of these ingredients have contributed to the establishment of the subject we now recognize as modern immunology.

The astute observations of Edward Jenner that recovery from cowpox protected against the grave effects of smallpox, together with his empirical immunization of James Phipps, laid the scientific basis of vaccination, an eighteenth-century validation of observations made in ancient China and of the risky practice of variolation (using directly the vesicle fluid from sufferers of smallpox).

It is apparent that the immune system evolved as a defence against infectious diseases in order to maintain the homeostasis of the organism. Clinical observations of individuals with congenital or acquired defects of their immune system strongly support this postulate. Furthermore, classical experiments performed with laboratory animals, resulting in controlled deletion and replacement of elements of the immune system further illustrate the basis of an efficient immune system. Humans or experimental animals who are immune-deficient suffer from a combination of serious, persistent, unusual, or recurrent microbial infections.

Many other aspects of the host contribute to preventing the entry of potentially damaging organisms. Thus, the integrity of the skin, the hostile environment in the gastrointestinal tract, substances such as lysozyme in the bodily secretions—all of which collectively form elements of *innate* immunity—provide excellent front-line defences against potential microbial invaders. The features, however, that set aside the established immune response, are its specificity, its memory, and its diversity—all aspects of an *adaptive immunity* (Table 1.1). These elements of adaptive immunity provide the basis whereby multiple entry of non-self components (i.e., microbes, proteins, chemicals—collectively termed antigens), will lead to *specific recognition* of each as separate non-self entities and the probable induction of a response against them. Most importantly, if a member of the original group of antigens is encountered again, it will be recognized specifically, and this second encounter will lead to an enhanced response. This implies that following the first encounter, a defined and predetermined perturbation occurred in the homeostasis of the organism and its immune system, which resulted in the generation of a 'memory' for that non-self substance. Following both the primary response and the memory-based secondary immune response—both of which have exquisite specificity for the exciting antigen—non-specific augmentation of the effects of the response occur which ultimately lead to the destruction or containment of the antigen. These augmenting effectors (recruited by and interacting with the specific immune factors) are substances such as complement and phagocytic cells (Fig. 1.1). The overall expression of these interactions results in the features of immune-induced inflammatory responses—the final common pathways for eliminating the antigens. Thus inflammation, when induced in a controlled and regulated manner, can be seen as the beneficial final pathway of an efficient immune response.

The cells responsible for the features of specificity, memory, and diversity

Table 1.1. Cells and soluble factors involved in innate and adaptive immune mechanisms

	Immunity	
Cells and factors	**Innate (natural, non-specific)**	**Adaptive (specific)**
Cells	Macrophages, monocytes, neutrophils, eosinophils, mast cells, platelets, 'natural killer' cells	T and B lymphocytes, antigen-presenting cells (APC)
Soluble factors	Complement, cytokines, lysozyme, interferons, acute phase proteins	Antibodies: IgM, IgG, IgA, IgD, and IgE; lymphokines
Other factors	Physical and mechanical barriers Genetic—species susceptibilities	Immunogenetics

Many of the cells and soluble factors of the innate and adaptive immune system interact and synergize in action against antigens, as expressed in forms of chronic and acute inflammation (protective and pathological).

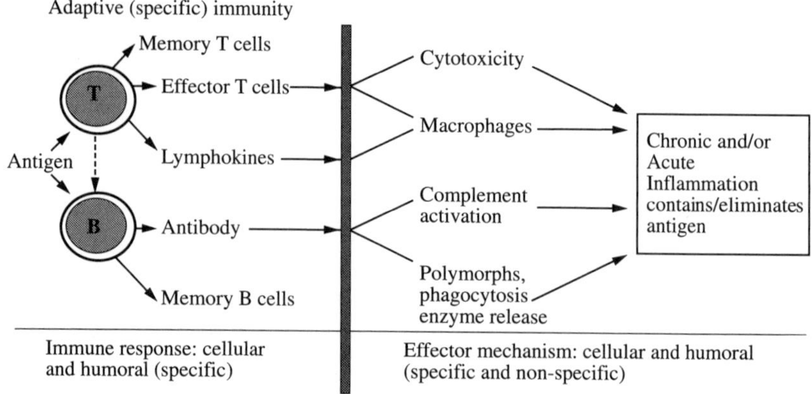

Fig. 1.1. Cells of the specific immune response responding to antigens. T and B lymphocytes and their secreted products recruit and interact with factors of innate immunity to destroy antigens.

of the immune response are the *lymphocytes*. They and their progeny produce molecules and recruit effectors which result in the expression of an immune response which can be conveniently defined at two levels: (1) *humoral immunity* which results in the generation of fluid phase antibodies which interact specifically with antigen; and (2) *cell-mediated immunity* (CMI) associated with and transferable by intact lymphoid cells. The central role of lymphocytes was demonstrated by classic experiments, which depleted animals of lymphocytes by various manœuvres, such as chronic thoracic duct drainage, surgical extirpation of lymphoid organs, and by transference of lymphoid cells. These experiments showed that lymphocytes contained the information for making antibody and for transferring the elements of cellular immunity as recognized by and embodied in phenomena, such as rejection of skin grafts, and killing of virus-infected cells which display viral antigens on their cell surfaces (Table 1.2).

Observations of rare immune deficiency states in man—such as the Di George syndrome—associated with congenital thymic aplasia, and of experimental surgical extirpation of the thymus in birds and mammals, led to the definition of a set of lymphocytes called thymic-dependent lymphocytes or T cells. The development, expression of receptors specific for antigens and the effector functions of T cells were dependent on an intact and functioning thymus. The athymic animals were also observed to have quantitatively significantly fewer lymphoid cells in blood and at various tissue sites, compared with the normal counterparts, and showed significant defects of cellular and humoral immunity (Table 1.2). These latter observations indicated that T lymphocytes represented the major lymphoid population in blood and also that although T cells were not

Table 1.2. The role of T and B Lymphocytes—the agents of specific (adaptive) immunity

T cells		**B cells (and derived plasma cells)**
Cell-mediated immunity (CMI)		**Humoral immunity (antibody)**
CMI responses		*Antibody responses*
Resistance to intracellular microbes		Neutralization
Rejection of transplant grafts (acute)		Cell lysis of microbes
Delayed type hypersensitivity		Opsonization
Contact dermatitis		Hyperacute graft rejection
Resistance to some tumours		Type I–III hypersensitivity
Effects of lymphocyte loss		
	CMI	*Humoral immunity*
1. Intact animal (no loss)	+++	+++
2. Loss of T cells		
• thymectomy	–	+
• Di George syndrome	–	+
3. Loss of B cells		
• bursectomy	++	–
• hypogammaglobulinaemia	+++	– (±)

directly involved in antibody synthesis they somehow affected cells responsible for antibody production. Birds were soon shown to have another discrete organ named the bursa of Fabricius, which was responsible for the development of another set of lymphocytes—termed B cells. Mammals do not possess a bursa, but the bone marrow (throughout life) and to some extent the fetal liver subserve similar functions in generating recognizable B lymphocytes. B cells and their progeny are responsible for the synthesis and secretion of antibodies.

Elegant *in vitro* experiments in the 1960s and 1970s clearly demonstrated that the early recognition events, involving the non-self antigens and the specific lymphocytes, required in most situations the interaction of cells of the mononuclear phagocytic system. Cells defined as belonging to this system include tissue macrophages, blood monocytes, circulating, and non-circulating tissue dendritic cells. It was demonstrated that these cells, at varying efficiencies, are able to present antigens in such a manner as to allow their recognition by lymphocytes and thus facilitate the triggering of the immune response. Such participating cells from the mononuclear phagocytic system, are now collectively termed *antigen-presenting cells* (APCs). Following the recognition of antigen by lymphocytes and the activation of the latter cells a series of events are set in motion, which ultimately result in the generation of the effector phases of the immune response associated with antibodies (humoral immunity) and effector T lymphocytes (CMI). The convenient descriptive separation of humoral immunity and CMI, and their association respectively with B cells and T cells, is clearly an over-simplification. As is apparent from Table 1.2, the two systems are to some extent interdependent. Thus, T lymphocytes are now seen as the pivotal cells in the recognition/early phase of all immune responses because, apart from providing the effector cells for CMI, they also provide *immunoregulatory T cells*, such as those providing 'help' for B cell synthesis of antibody (see later), and other cells involved in the functional regulation of immune responses. Furthermore, recent experiments have indicated that B cells, apart from antibody production, are able to modulate T cell responses as well as function as APC for T cells.

1.2 Overview of the immune system

1.2.1 Clusters of differentiation (CD) molecules and monoclonal antibodies (MABs)

Hybridoma biotechnology as originally described by Köhler and Milstein in 1975 (see Chapter 9, p. 179.) has produced many monoclonal antibodies (MABs). The latter have been employed as tools to dissect the complexities and characterize the nature of the molecules and cells within the immune system. Such reagents have contributed significantly to defining leucocyte development, and lymphocyte physiology and immunopathology. MABs, by international workshop agreement, have been placed into groupings according to their reactions with specific antigens—termed clusters of differentiation (CD). These antigens representing proteins, glycoproteins, and glycolipids have been in most cases partially characterized. Documented below are some selected examples of CD groupings which should prove useful in subsequent sections of this and other chapters.

CD defines the *antigen*, generally of known molecular weight (shown as kilodaltons (kDa)), against which a series of MABs have been derived. Currently, by common usage, the antibodies against the defined CD antigens, are also now referred to as the CD antibodies (grouping together various synonymous reagents produced by different researchers and companies).

Outline of some selected CD specificities

CD1—a group of antigens (43–49 kDa) detected on and restricted to normal lymphocytes within the thymus (i.e., thymocytes). Some of these antigens, detected by 'CD1-antibodies' (synonyms: OKT6, Leu 6), can also be demonstrated on Langerhans cells, i.e., APC cells of skin and associated pathological cells found in the histiocytosis X complex.

CD2—an antigen (~ 50 kDa) present on all normal T lymphocytes, i.e., a pan-T cell marker, it is also detectable on a population of morphologically defined large granular lymphocytes (LGL), which have demonstrable 'natural killer' (NK) cell function (see Section 1.5.3). The CD2 antigen functions as the receptor (also named lymphocyte functioning antigen 2 (LFA2)) for sheep erythrocytes, the basis of the old E rosette assay for demonstrating T cells.

CD3—defines a multimolecular antigen complex (including 19, 21, 26 kDa molecules) restricted to T lymphocytes (synonyms: OKT3, UCHT1, Leu 4). The CD3 molecules are closely associated on the T cell membrane with the antigen-specific T cell receptor molecule Ti. The complex is often referred to as CD3/Ti, or T3/Ti complex or abbreviated as TCR.

CD4—the 55 kDa antigen is detected on the major subset of peripheral T lymphocytes—the *T helper/inducer subset*. Also, the CD4 antigen, which is known to function as a receptor for the human immunodeficiency virus (HIV) associated with AIDS (see Chapter 8), forms an integral part of the membrane of monocyte-macrophage cells (synonyms: OKT4, Leu 3). In addition, CD4 is expressed on developing thymocytes located within the thymus.

CD5—another pan-T cell antigen but also found on a rare subset of normal B cells and commonly on certain neoplastic B cell clones of chronic lymphocytic leukaemia and non-Hodgkins lymphoma. CD5-expressing B cells may have an important role to play in the production of autoantibodies in autoimmune disorders (see Section 1.6.2 and Chapter 8).

CD8—an antigen detected on a subset of peripheral T lymphocytes—*T suppressor/cytotoxic cells* (synonyms: Leu 2a, OKT8). CD8 is also expressed on developing thymocytes.

CD10—a 100 kDa molecule called the common acute lymphoblastic leukaemia antigen (CALLA) defined originally on the pathological leukaemic cells from which it was first isolated, and now known to represent an antigen associated with early B lymphocyte development. It is detectable also on granulocytes, renal, and gastrointestinal epithelium.

CD11—a series of antigens (150–180 kDa) defining a family of adhesion molecules associated with cell to cell interactions and functions, and called varying names, such as lymphocyte functioning antigen 1 (LFA1). The CD11 series is detectable on a wide spectrum of leucocytes, including monocytes, granulocytes, and subsets of T and B cells.

CD14—an antigen (50–55 kDa) known to be specifically expressed on the membrane of blood monocytes, although it can be detected in the cytoplasm of granulocytes.

CD15—antigen (50–180 kDa) present on the myeloid-monocytic series of cells, on some epithelial cells and corresponding carcinomas, as well as on the Reed–Sternberg cells associated with Hodgkin's disease (synonym: Leu M1).

CD16—defines an antigen on the cell membrane (50–60 kDa) which functionally interacts at low affinity with the Fc portion of the IgG class of immunoglobulins (see Section 1.3.2). CD16 is located on polymorphs, eosinophils, NK cells, and lymphokine activated killer (LAK) cells within the morphologically defined LGL population. Such cells are currently being investigated in strategies of adoptive immunotherapy of cancer (see Chapter 7).

CD19—defines an antigen restricted to the B lymphocyte lineage, i.e., is a pan-B cell antigen, and is believed to be involved in B cell differentiation. MABs to CD19 are extremely useful for specific qualitative and quantitative enumeration of B cells.

CD21—defines an antigen (140 kDa) on some B cells and APC cells of the lymph node termed dendritic reticulum cells. The CD21 antigen is also known to function as a receptor for the Epstein–Barr virus. Some epithelial cells, e.g., epithelium of the uterine cervix have been demonstrated to express CD21. CD21 is known to be a functional receptor for fragments of activated complement termed C3d (see Section 1.5.1) and is referred to as CR2.

CD25—this antigen (50–55 kDa) defines a so-called 'activation antigen marker' present on activated T cells, following their specific interaction with antigens, or non-specific mitogenic stimuli (synonyms: interleukin-2 (IL-2) receptor and TAC antigen). In pathological states CD25 is associated with certain leukaemias and lymphomas. Physiologically, the T cell-derived lymphokine IL-2 (see Section 1.4.1) binds specifically to CD25, and is an important signal for T cell activation and proliferation in CMI, and in T cell regulatory mechanisms.

CD45—defines antigens of differing molecular weights (180–220 kDa) found on leucocytes (synonym: leucocyte common antigen, LCA) characterizing cells of leucocyte origin. Diagnostically, the CD45 specificity contributes greatly in the differential diagnosis of anaplastic cancers (e.g., lymphoma versus carcinoma) (see Chapter 9).

CD56—an antigen (~ 220 kDa) expressed on most NK cells and a subset of T cells which exhibit cytotoxic function (synonyms: NKH-1, Leu 19). CD56 is also recognized to be an iso-form of a neural intercellular adhesion molecule called N-CAM.

The above brief summary of some important CDs is mainly restricted to their expression on cells, i.e., their *phenotypic* demonstration. The exploitation of phenotypes to enumerate cell numbers and subsets, cell development, and functional properties will be illustrated throughout this text. It is to be appreciated that the molecules defined by the CDs are assumed to have specific biological functions associated with the cells possessing them; these functional aspects of CDs are only now becoming clearer. Their elucidation has been greatly helped by exploiting molecular biological techniques, allowing isolation and cloning of genes encoding the CDs, and the subsequent transfection, i.e., direct DNA insertion—incorporation and expression of the 'genes' and their encoded products in *in vitro* cell lines (see Chapter 9). Thus, one of the *in vivo* biological roles of the T cell CD4 antigen is apparently to interact with molecules associated with expressed MHC (major histocompatability complex—Section 1.3.1) gene products on APC. Other less strong evidence also suggests the CD4 antigen may function as a growth factor receptor for certain cytokines (i.e., soluble secreted polypeptides from various cells types). Similarly, the CD3 molecular complex has been defined as playing an important role in signal transduction from the CD3/Ti receptor complex on the cell surface through the cell membrane to the cell cytosol and ultimately to the nucleus of the T cell. This 'signal transduction' represents critical biochemical information which flows from the interaction of the 'foreign antigen complex' with the T cell membrane antigen receptor to ultimately result in effector CMI reactions which will destroy or contain the foreign antigen. Many steps in this transduction process, as yet, are ill defined. Nevertheless, the recent characterization of patients with rare deficiencies associated with lack of expression of parts of the CD3 complex, supports the proposed functions.

At the time of writing, in excess of 70 CD antigens have been defined and are internationally recognized, but in the vast majority of cases, their true functional roles are far from established; nevertheless, they are still invaluable for the phenotyping of cells.

1.2.2 Central and peripheral lymphoid organs

The *anatomical network* comprising the immune system is depicted in Figs 1.2 and 1.3. Some features of the human lymphoid system are described below.

Thymus

This central lymphoid organ, located in the upper anterior mediastinum in humans, is known to be the primary site for the development of T lymphocytes from immigrant bone marrow lymphoid stem cells, which migrate into the thymus from as early as 8 weeks of gestation. The inductive factors of the thymus responsible for the differentiation of stem cells

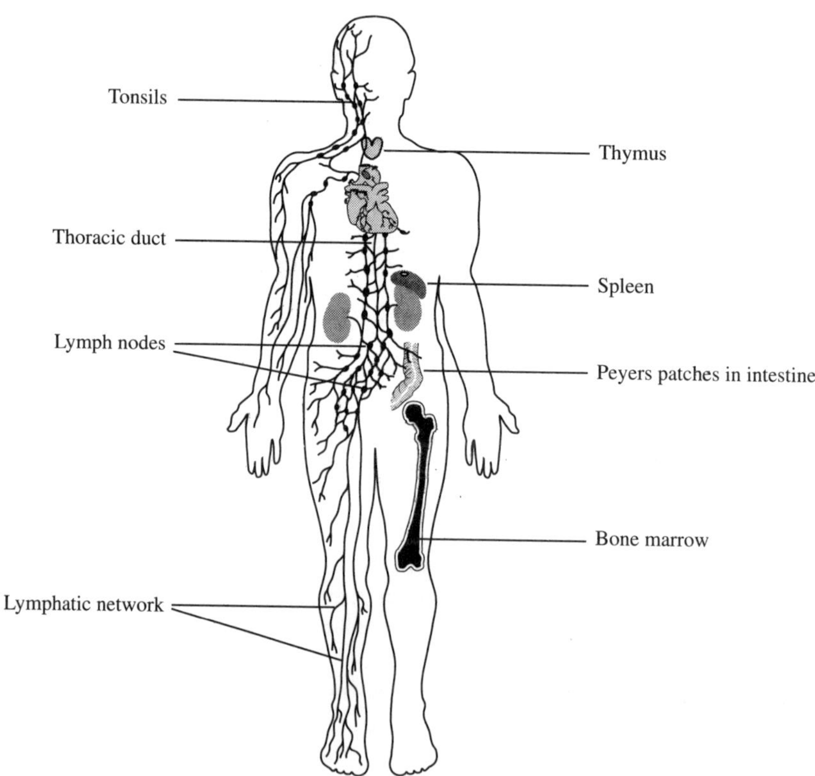

Fig. 1.2. The human lymphoid system. T and B lymphocytes can be defined in compartments within the tissue as well as undergoing continuous recirculation between lymphatics, blood, and lymphoid organs. Thymus and bone marrow function as central (primary) organs for development of T and B cells.

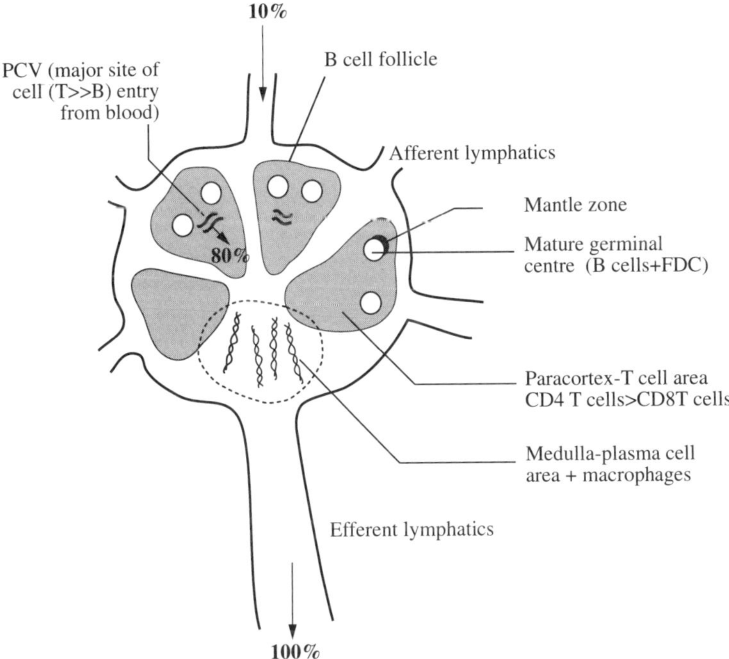

Fig. 1.3 Organization of the lymph node structure facilitates entry of antigen and its specific interaction with the appropriate T and B cells. PCV, post-capillary venule; FDC, follicular dendritic (antigen-presenting) cell; %, estimate of lymphocyte traffic. > greater than; ≫ substantially greater than.

to thymic lymphocytes (thymocytes) include a number of small polypeptide hormones. Several such hormones have been isolated, including thymosin (~ 12 kDa) and thymopoietin (~ 7 kDa). Organ culture experiments have clearly indicated that direct cell-to-cell contact between the bone marrow-derived cells and the mesenchymal/stromal, dendritic, and epithelial elements of the thymus also are necessary for normal cell proliferation and differentiation.

A scheme for thymocyte development is shown in Fig. 1.4, indicating recognized T cell-associated CD antigens. These CD differentiation antigens are acquired at various stages within the thymus, the most undifferentiated cells being found in the outer cortex and the most mature in the medulla. From the medulla a small percentage of cells migrate out of the thymus, to become the antigen-responsive immunocompetent T lymphocytes recognized in the periphery, i.e., secondary lymphoid T cell compartments. Thus, peripheral T cells are found in the paracortex of lymph nodes (Fig. 1.3), the white pulp of the spleen, as the major population of

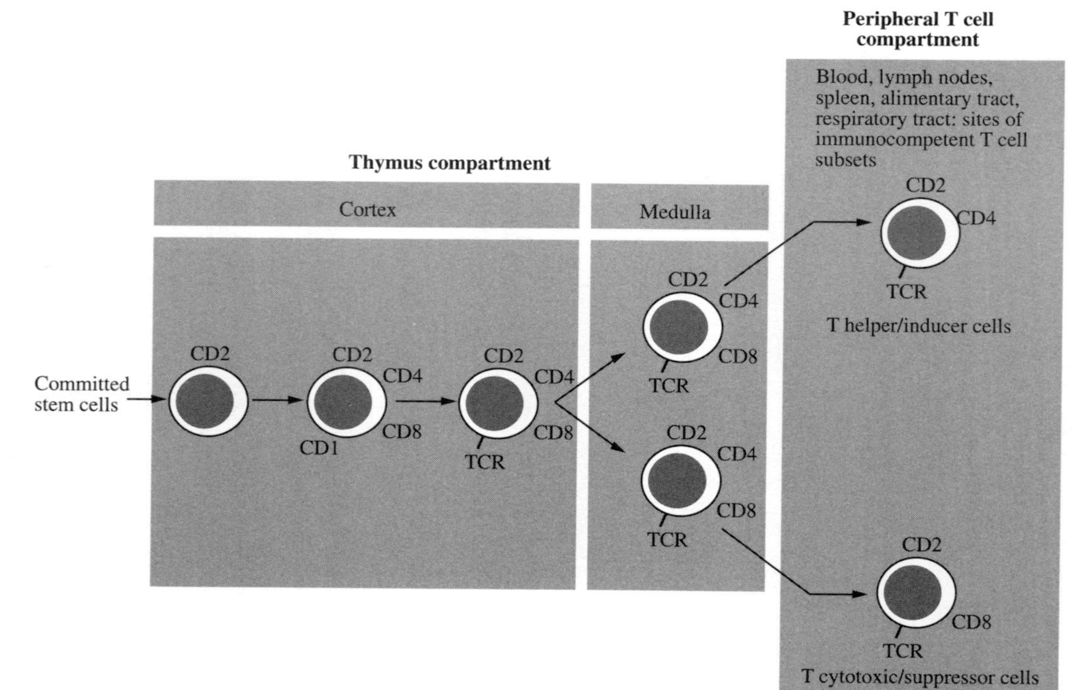

Fig. 1.4. T cell development within the thymus and emergent T cells in the peripheral compartment. CD, cluster of differentiation antigen; TCR, T cell antigen receptor (CD3/Ti complex).

lymphocytes in blood, and as intraepithelial and lamina propria T cells, and as lymphoid aggregrates in the alimentary tract and other mucosal sites.

It has been well established that both massive proliferation and death of cells occurs in the thymus. These events have been demonstrated by classic histological methods as well as by labelling cells with radioisotopes and following the fate of labelled cells. Experiments on mice have demonstrated that within the thymus more than 10^8 lymphocytes are produced per day, but only about 10^6 cells are exported to the periphery. Hence, less than 10 per cent of the cells produced within the organ survive and exit from the gland. This apparent 'mysterious' behaviour within the thymus has recently begun to be unravelled by modern cellular and molecular biological techniques.

The *raison d'être* of the thymus seems to be two-fold: (1) The generation and the selective maturation of single $CD4^+$ and $CD8^+$ immunocompetent cells respectively which exit from the thymus. The cells possess specific antigen receptor complexes (TCRs) which will recognize a vast array of potential foreign antigens—complexed with self MHC (major histocompatibility complex) molecules (see Section 1.3.1)—to mount an efficient immune response. (2) To destroy within the thymus, developing cells which during proliferation and differentiation develop TCRs with the potential to react strongly solely against self antigens (rather than against foreign antigen + self MHC). Intrathymic destruction of such cells is seen as a crucial mechanism in the development of self tolerance and thus a lack of pathological responses to self antigens, as occurs in autoimmunity (Section 1.6.2).

The first category (1) is thought to occur by a process termed *positive selection*. Developing cortical thymocytes (possessing both CD4 and CD8) with TCR binding to particular molecules on thymic epithelial cells (with self antigens including self MHC) are *selected* for survival. The future TCR recognition of foreign antigens (outside the thymus) by these cells will also require them to 'see' the self molecules responsible for their survival. Thymocytes which do not bind to the self molecules at this stage of development undergo apoptosis (a process of programmed cell death). There is strong experimental evidence indicating that for (2) a process of *negative selection* occurs, whereby cells now with strong binding TCRs for self molecules (perhaps encountered at the cortico-medullary junction) are deleted, again via the process of apoptosis. The CD4 and CD8 molecules on thymocytes are believed to play direct and contributory roles in the processes of positive and negative selection—but these mechanisms require more clarification.

Thus, the mature T cells trafficking from the thymus are cell populations with the properties of: (i) mainly *unresponsiveness* to self antigens alone (mainly self MHC); (ii) the ability to react to MHC antigen of other members of the species (the basis of recognition of MHC antigens in transplantation, leading to acute rejection); and (iii) the ability to react with foreign antigen, associated with self MHC (a phenomenon termed MHC restriction). This massive cell proliferation will generate many different families of cells (clones) with TCR to recognize and interact with the many millions of antigens which may be encountered in life. The price of such diversity could be the development of TCRs with anti-self specificity. Such clones, however, would be largely (if not totally) deleted in the massive cell death phenomenon in the thymus.

Bursa—bursa equivalents

B lymphopoeisis, like T lymphopoeisis, takes place in a primary lymphoid organ. In birds, a discrete organ found near the cloaca—the bursa of Fabricius—has been shown to be responsible for the development of B cells from bone marrow lymphoid stem cell precursors. In mammals, no bursa exists, but there is experimental evidence that the bone marrow and the fetal yolk sac and liver subserve a similar function. Modern techniques using monoclonal antibodies and radionuclide tracing have clearly defined differentiation pathways of B cell development (see Fig. 1.5)—analogous to T cells in the thymic environment.

A feature common to both T and B primary organs is that the cells in their early development in those sites are relatively immuno-incompetent; they will not react positively and generate immune responses against classic non-self antigens. Immuno-competent T and B lymphocytes, by contrast, are found in the so-called secondary lymphoid organs and other sites.

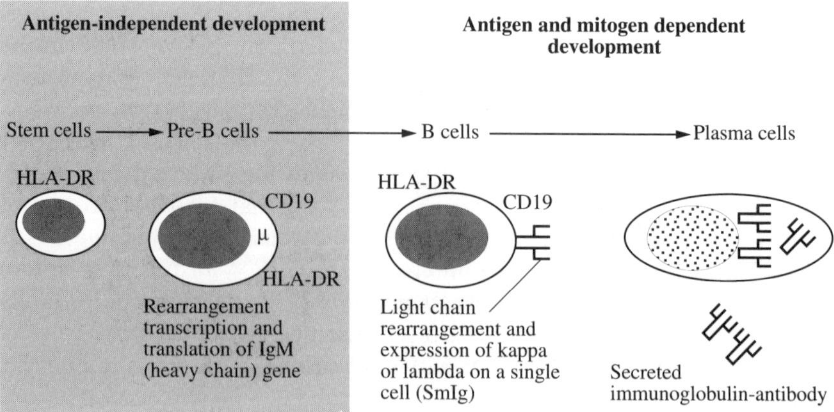

Fig. 1.5. B lymphocyte development. Surface membrane immunoglobulin (smIg) on the B cell functions as the antigen-specific receptor.

Secondary lymphoid organs

The common feature of all these sites, i.e., lymph nodes, spleen, tonsils, etc., is that T and B cells can be found in fairly identifiable compartments and are closely juxtaposed anatomically to members of the APC family. Figure 1.3 shows a cross-section of a lymph node with the predominant collection of T cells in the paracortex and B cells in the follicular areas. Plasma cells, which are derived from B cells and secrete antibody molecules, can be found in the medullary region. In all of these areas of the node, appropriate APCs can be demonstrated.

The lymphatic network—recirculation pathways

The lymphoid cells detectable in a blood differential count consist of T cells (~ 50–90 per cent), B cells (~ 5–15 per cent), and a minor population (~ 1–10 per cent) of the large granular lymphocytes (LGL) which contain the natural killer (NK) cells. The blood T and B cells enter the substance of lymph nodes through the post-capillary venules. The cells then traffic through the respective T and B areas of the node and together with a smaller percentage of cells, which enter via the afferent lymphatics, leave the node via the efferent lymphatics. Figure 1.3 shows this traffic, based on experiments using fine needle cannulation of the lymphatics and blood vessels. Ultimately, the lymphatics empty into the blood system where the thoracic duct joins the left subclavian vein and bloodstream, from whence the lymphocytes recirculate.

The lymphatics, which also transport antigens in solution or associated with APC in the lymph as well as facilitating the recirculation of lymphocytes, provide a most efficient system for immune cells to encounter and interact with non-self antigens irrespective of where such antigens have managed to breach the integrity of the organism.

The concept of specificity within the immune system coupled with its evident ability to react against thousands/millions of different antigens is best explained and crystallized in the *clonal selection theory* of immunology. This original concept, elaborated in various forms by Burnet, Jerne, and Talmage to explain antibody production, is now equally applied to T lymphocyte responses.

1.2.3 Clonal selection

Apart from its *specificity* and *memory*, the other striking feature of the immune system is its *diversity*. The complement of T and B lymphocytes within an individual can react to a great number (calculated to be in excess of one million) of non-self antigens. How does such enormous diversity come about and how is it harmonized with the salient features of immunological specificity and memory? These properties have become comprehensible

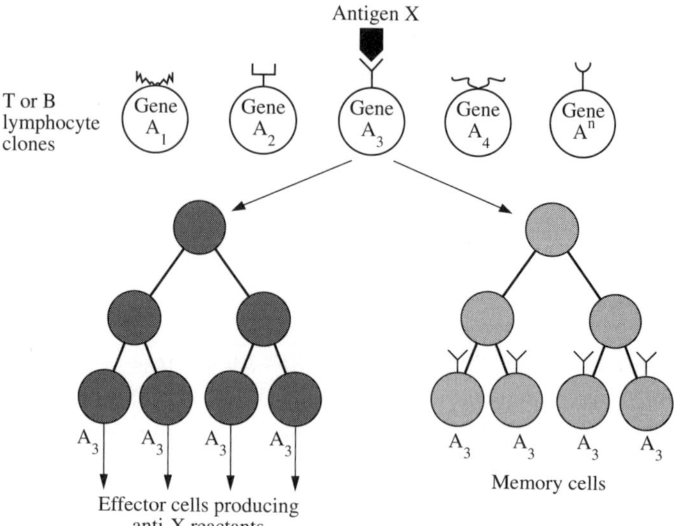

Fig. 1.6. Clonal selection. Antigen X selects and interacts with the clone expressing the 'best fit' (complementarity) receptor. The clone responds by differentiation–proliferation to generate anti-X effector and memory cells.

and explicable on the basis of the clonal selection theory. Figure 1.6 represents the essence of the theory, the basis of which is as follows:

1. A lymphocyte and its identical progeny, termed *a clone*, (identical with respect to their genes) possess on their cell membranes receptors with specific binding sites for only one or a very limited number of antigenic determinants. The number of cells comprising a single clone (e.g., clone A_3) have been calculated as ranging from 10^3 to 10^5 in the B and T cell compartments. Estimates of the total number of lymphocytes in man suggest greater than 10^{14} cells. Thus with simple arithmetical analysis, in excess of 10^6 different (A_1, A_2, . . . A^n) clones are possible. The mechanisms of receptor specificity for antigen are explained in terms of the genetics and molecular events that occur during the development of B and T cells and are outlined in the sections on B and T cells (see Section 1.3).

2. Implicit in the clonal selection theory is the idea that the specificity of a clone antedates any experience or encounter with classical non-self antigens, i.e., lymphocyte clones possess specific receptors, each precommitted to a single antigen. Thus, ultimately, when antigen is encountered, *selection* of a precommitted clone with the 'best fitting receptor' for that antigen occurs.

From Fig. 1.6, the shape of the receptor expressed on the surface of

A_3 gives the basis of the *specificity*. The events following receptor-antigen interaction involve cell proliferation and differentiation, resulting in the exponential expansion of the responding clone, some of the clone members proceeding to end-stage effector cells, which will act against the inciting antigen. In the case of B cell clones, some of the cells differentiate into plasma cells and secrete antibodies with the same specificity as that expressed by the B cell receptor originally selected by the antigen. Similarly, for CMI some T cells differentiate into effector cells, such as cytotoxic T cells. It is noteworthy that with clonal expansion not all the progeny become end-stage effectors. Some reach an intermediate point of differentiation and proliferation, and such cells form the cellular basis for the immunological property of *memory*. Thus, if the same antigen is encountered on a subsequent occasion, the memory bank of cells undergoes a quantitatively greater response against the antigen (see also Fig. 1.10). Note that clonal expansion gives four memory cells each with the specific A_3 receptor for antigen compared with only one cell in the original primary response. Furthermore, the clonal expansion events also qualitatively result in changes in the affinity (strength of binding) of the lymphocyte receptor for antigen—although maintaining the same specificity.

Most experimental evidence, to date, supports the tenets of the clonal selection theory. Suicide experiments using high dose radiolabelled antigens have resulted in radiation deletion of specific clones; re-challenge with the same antigen gives no response, yet challenge with a different antigen elicits an appropriate response. Recent experiments have indicated that certain sites, such as the germinal centres of lymph nodes, provide the appropriate microenvironment for generating 'memory' B lymphocytes and for long-term retention of small amounts of antigen on specialized APC within the germinal centre.

Summary of clonal selection theory

Immunocompetent lymphocytes bear glycoprotein receptors on their cell membranes. Lymphocytes undergoing activation and differentiation retain the same specificity of their receptors for antigens as that of their progenitors. Thus, in the case of the B lymphocyte, its antibody receptor V region specificity (see Section 1.3.2) is the same as the binding specificity of antibodies secreted from plasma cells derived from the B cells. Each immunocompetent lymphocyte (representing a member of a clone) bears receptors of unique specificity when compared with receptors on a lymphocytes from another clone.

1.2.4 Immunogens, antigens, and adjuvants

The term *immunogen* is used to denote substances which have the property of inducing detectable immune responses when introduced into an animal.

The term antigen strictly defines substances that will react with preformed immune effector molecules but that will not necessarily induce the production of such immune effectors. All immunogens can be antigens but the converse is not always true. Through imprecise usage over many years the term immunogen and antigen are now often used interchangeably. Large proteins are usually the most efficient antigens but polysaccharides, synthetic polypeptides, and simple polymers can also be antigenic. Pure nucleic acids have been shown experimentally to be non-immunogenic, yet it is known that humans and other animals can produce, in old age and in autoimmune disorders, antibodies that will react with nucleic acids. Hence, patients with systemic lupus erythematosus (SLE) may have antibodies against different nucleic acids, including those reacting with double-stranded DNA. It may be that antibodies arise against large nucleoproteins (or cross-reacting substances) and that some antibodies have the ability to react specifically with the associated nucleic acid.

There are several well-defined properties of molecules which render them good immunogens. Foremost of these properties is their *'foreignness'*, which the immune system discriminates from self. The size of the molecule is important and as a generalization, molecules more than 10 kDa tend to be strongly antigenic, especially if they are polypeptides. The actual *genetic background* of the animal exposed to a non-self substance, may dictate whether the substance functions as an antigen. Careful experiments with inbred strains of mice, rats, and guinea pigs have clearly documented the existence of so-called *immune response genes*, which determine whether an introduced non-self substance will function as an antigen in the animal. The immune response gene effect has most often been shown to be expressed as an autosomal dominant trait.

The apparent antigenicity of a substance will also depend on the *dose* and its *route* of administration to the animal. In fact, in some situations a non-self substance known to be extremely antigenic can fail to elicit an immune response. This effect is produced by manœuvres, such as intravenous injection of very small or very large doses of antigen, i.e., either side of the standard antigenic dose. In the latter, a definite negative influence is exerted on the immune system such that a *tolerant* state (acquired immunological tolerance) is induced to that foreign antigen.

Classic experiments by Landsteiner defined the properties of substances called *haptens*. These are molecules (usually very small) which by themselves are unable to induce an immune response, i.e., function as antigens/immunogens. Nevertheless, they are capable of being recognized by and interacting with, antibodies or effector T cells induced by another means. The experimental method of inducing the immune response is usually to link the small hapten to a larger carrier molecule—this provides the necessary information for the combined molecule to be recognized as an antigen. In general terms, it has been demonstrated that the 'carrier' molecules are recognized by T cells and that the antibodies produced by the B cells will recognize and bind the hapten. The study of 'haptenization' of large molecules, provides an explanation of how diverse substances, including very small metallic ions (e.g., nickel), anaesthetic gases, such as halothane, and antibodies, such as penicillin can induce, in individuals of the appropriate genetic background demonstrable immune responses, often of a pathological type. It is suggested that the small molecules complex to normal readily accessible self proteins, such as albumin and pre-albumin (which are widely distributed extra- and intravascularly). The complexing presents 'altered' self-determinants which can appear as non-self to immune cells and thus induce humoral and cell-mediated responses, some of which are directed to the haptens of the complex.

Concept of complementarity

The interaction of antigen with antibody or with the specific receptor on the membrane of T and B lymphocytes is often expressed in terms of a 'lock and key' interaction. It should best be thought of in terms of the overall three-dimensional shape, which is recognized by the receptor or antibody regions which interact with the complementary shape of the antigen. The affinity of binding of the specific immune elements with the antigen can be though of in terms of their degree of closeness of fit or complementarity. Apparent antigen *cross-reactions* may thus be accounted for in regard to overall complementarity rather than their likeness in terms of overall charge or size. Thus, well-documented cross-reactions, such as seen with certain streptococcal antigens that induce antibodies which can cross-react and bind to other very dissimilar (in terms of size and charge) human cardiac antigens, result from the closeness in overall shape of the two molecules and their complementarity with the antibody's '*antigen combining regions*' (or complementarity determining regions, CDR).

A further consequence of considering the overall shape of antigens and the corresponding binding regions of antibodies and lymphocyte receptors is the realization that, even though antigens may be very large molecules, it is only a few sites (usually accessible surface sites) of a large folded protein structure that are recognized by B lymphocytes and antibodies. The sites are termed the *antigenic determinants* or *epitopes* of the antigen molecule. It is calculated that four to six amino acids or sugar residues may contribute to an epitope of a protein or polysaccharide antigen respectively. T lymphocytes appear not to recognize native conformational (folded) protein antigen epitopes as described for B lymphocytes. Instead, they recognize peptide fragments of antigens, which undergo significant '*processing*' usually within APC.

A single, large antigen, therefore, may induce both T and B cell responses, usually elicited to different epitopes on the same molecule. Furthermore, it appears that the immune response to the great majority of antigens requires the dual function of T and B cells. In fact, the B cell antibody response (for optimal results) requires T cell recognition of the same molecule—albeit different epitopes—to provide 'help' for an efficient antibody response. These types of antigens are often referred to as *thymus (T cell)-dependent antigens*. Contrastingly, there is a group of substances termed thymus-independent (TI) antigens, which have the property of eliciting B lymphocyte and antibody responses with minimal requirement for T cell involvement. Such TI antigens are exemplified by bacterial polysaccharides, which have the structural feature of many identical repeating molecules and epitopes.

The recent advances in the isolation and molecular cloning of genes have led to the possibility of generating large amounts of pure antigens for vaccination programmes. This is particularly so in the case of complex microbial antigens. Parasites, like those causing malaria or schistosomiasis, are very complex organisms with potentially hundreds of epitopes, some of which may induce protective immune responses. Researchers, using molecular biological techniques, are now defining and cloning specific genes, to produce a single or a few dominant antigens and their epitopes in the hope of generating vaccines to the latter in order to combat such pandemic infections. Furthermore, the acquired knowledge concerning the generation of processed peptides as antigens is also resulting in attempts to synthesize tailor-made peptide antigens for vaccination programmes. Both approaches, namely those of gene cloning and peptide synthesis, are currently being employed in the fight against AIDS, seeking to define and produce non-infectious peptide antigens of HIV to use in possible vaccination programmes.

Adjuvants represent a wide range of compounds which act in a non-specific immunostimulatory fashion to enhance the immunogenicity/antigenicity of weak antigens. The classical adjuvant is *Freund's complete adjuvant* (FCA), which is a combination of mycobacterial products, organic oils, and a detergent. FCA is commonly mixed with a solution of antigen, to form an injectable emulsion. The resultant antigen-adjuvant complex is a very potent stimulator of the immune response. FCA, however, is so potent that it is not used in man as it induces extensive granulomatous reactions at the injection site. Adjuvants, in general, have been shown experimentally to non-specifically increase the action of macrophages and other APCs and to enhance T and B lymphocyte functions.

In humans, the most commonly used adjuvants are aluminium compounds (alums), which form precipitates with antigens in common usage, such as tetanus toxoid and diphtheria toxoids. Newer adjuvants are being evaluated for use in man, especially those designed for increasing the antigenicity of synthetic peptides, and the newer DNA recombinant antigens. Two good examples of these newer adjuvants are muramyl dipeptide (MDP) and the so-called immunostimulatory complex (ISCOM). MDP represents a relatively non-toxic extract of mycobacterial membranes; ISCOM is composed of a glycoside extracted from the bark of an Amazonian tree which readily forms micelles containing entrapped peptide or polypeptide antigens, to form potent immunostimulatory complexes. It is hoped these newer adjuvants together with the new recombinant antigens, may contribute to the production of new and effective vaccines to various viruses, bacteria, and parasites.

1.3 Recognition elements, cells, and receptor molecules

1.3.1 Major histocompatibility complex (MHC)

The major histocompatibility complex (MHC) defines a discrete, chromosomally assigned region, where genes are located which encode, in their nucleotide bases, the information for the production of molecules (glycoproteins) which are expressed phenotypically on and in cells. The MHC of humans is located on the short arm of chromosome 6, and in mice on chromosome 17. Located within the MHC region are discrete loci (points) of defined genes. The classic products of human MHC genes are the glycoproteins—the human leucocyte antigens (HLA)—so-called due to the original demonstration of the ·products on leucocytes. Other genes are found within the MHC encoding for non-HLA glycoproteins. Figure 1.7 outlines the events from the level of the genes to the cell expression of HLA (some texts will also use the term MHC antigens to define the HLA).

The classical HLAs are termed class I and class II as are the corresponding

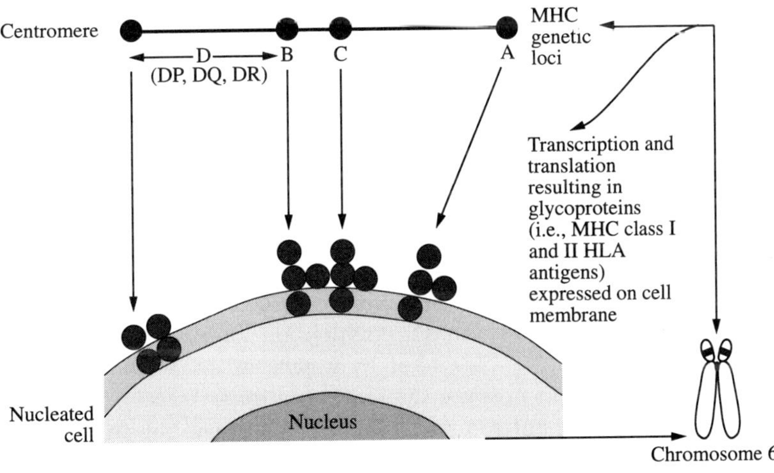

Fig. 1.7. The human major histocompatibility complex (MHC) and expressed human leucocyle antigens (HLA) at the cell membrane.

MHC gene loci; also found in the MHC region are other gene-encoding products which are designated class III antigens. Recently, the genes encoding some important cytokines, namely tumour necrosis factor (TNF) α and β also have been mapped in the human MHC region, between the B and D loci (see Chapter 2). The class I loci A, B, C encodes the HLA A, B, C antigens. In the near future the class I map and associated antigens will certainly be expanded. The class II loci (DR, DQ, and DP) encode the classical class II antigens termed HLA-DR, DQ, and DP. The summation of these loci is also referred to as the D region; corresponding antigens in rodents are called Ia. Further gene mapping experiments have documented a DZ/DO gene but the gene is not associated with defined and expressed glycoproteins on cells—such non-expressed genes are termed pseudogenes.

The classical MHCI and II genes represent a good example of an *allelic system*, i.e., within a species many alternative forms of a particular gene and its product are found within different members of the species. Thus, one individual may have a class I gene in locus A numbered as 2 which encodes for HLA-A2, whilst another individual will have a gene A10 and its product designated as HLA-A10. Currently, in excess of 20 alleles have been found in A, with more than 40 in B, 8 in C, 16 in DR, 3 in DQ, and 6 in DP. These different alleles are likely to increase in number with the use of refined methods of defining genes and their products (see Chapter 2).

The assigning of and analyses of HLA class I and II antigen specificity is based on a combination of serological (antibody) and cellular assays. More recently, DNA analyses, using restriction fragment length polymorphism (RFLP) and DNA hybridization techniques, have been performed. The allelic differences in the genes are due to minor variations in nucleotide base sequences, resulting in minor changes in the corresponding amino acid sequence (and associated conformational changes), in particular regions of the HLA glycoprotein. Apart from the subtle differences mentioned above, the overall form of HLA class I and class II products can be determined and are shown diagramatically in Fig. 1.8. The figure illustrates the concepts of 'domains'; that is, segments of the protein where defined lengths and sequences of amino acids can be seen as folding into a particular three-dimensional conformation. The HLA class I antigen, therefore, has $\alpha1$, $\alpha2$, and $\alpha3$ domains, which on the cell membrane are almost always associated with the small polypeptide called $\beta2$ microglobulin ($\beta2$M). The latter is not encoded for by a gene in the MHC, and in man the $\beta2$M gene is on chromosome 15. The evolutionary reason for the close association of class I antigen with $\beta2$M is not clear but functionally it appears to be necessary for the full expression of the HLA class I. The HLA class I antigen molecules are thus composed of two chains, designated α and β, although α is the true class I chain. Contrastingly, both chains

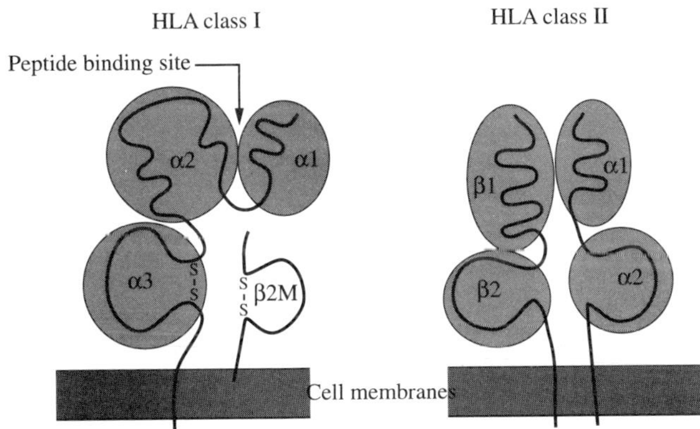

Fig. 1.8. HLA class I (with associated peptide binding site) and class II molecules expressed at the cell membrane. β2M, β2 microglobulin; α1, β1 denote domain units; S– S, disulphide bonds.

of the HLA class II antigens, termed α and β, are coded for by MHC genes.

The many alleles within the MHC genes, together with the potential for many differing combinations of A, B, C, DR, DQ, and DP, lead to a system which can also be defined as very *polymorphic*. The collection of MHC genes on a single chromosome is termed the *haplotype*; the *genotype* is determined by the paternal and maternal chromosomes. The inheritance of the MHC genes follows classic Mendelian patterns (see Chapter 2).

Linkage disequilibrium defines the situation where certain MHC genes are found associated together (linked) on a chromosome at a frequency far in excess of the predicted/expected occurence of these genes associating, if the association events were a completely random process through evolutionary time. The occurrence of linkage disequilibrium suggests, from an evolutionary perspective, some selective advantage to the organism for such a non-random association. Alternatively, the behaviour of the organisms may have been such as to minimize random selection, e.g., by manœuvres such as intensive inbreeding—which is clearly not the case in most examples of human evolution. The effects of linkage disequilibrium are further discussed in the chapters on transplantation (Chapter 2) and on autoimmunity (Chapter 8).

What is the role of the MHC genes and their products? The answers have come from several sources: (i) A careful documentation of the sites where the HLA class I and class II antigens are located; (ii) classical and elegant animal experiments, particularly in the 1970s; and (iii) recent biochemical and molecular biological experiments resulting in the isolation of MHC genes, their amino acid sequencing and X-ray crystallographic appearance, and analyses of intact MHC antigens.

By using MABs to the overall structures (non-polymorphic framework molecules) of class I and class II antigens, researchers have documented their distribution on cells. Class I antigens are ubiquitous whilst class II (in normal situations) can be seen to be restricted and expressed on cells intimately involved in the immune response, i.e., B lymphocytes, APC, and activated T cells. Cells bearing class II antigens also express class I antigens.

The classic experiments of Zinkernagel and Doherty and others in the 1970s demonstrated that for T cells to recognize an antigen, the antigen had to be complexed with the self MHC product, the phenomenon being termed MHC restriction (see the sections on the thymus, p. 10 and T cells, p. 33). Recent biochemical and molecular biological experiments have shown that protein antigens which complex with self MHC proteins, are commonly partially degraded antigen fragments, i.e., peptides of various sizes from the native molecule generated within APC. Recent X-ray crystallographic evidence has produced the first ever images of an MHC class I product—HLA class I antigen with a bound peptide, the binding site being associated with conformational sites and amino acids found in the $\alpha 1$ and $\alpha 2$ domains (see Fig. 1.8).

What then are the functions of the MHC? It is clear, from biological and evolutionary evidence that the MHC genes and their products did not evolve and persist just to frustrate transplant surgeons! The true physiological functions of the MHC in man and animals can be summarized as follows.

Physiological role of MHC

1. MHC molecules, by combining with peptide fragments (antigens), result in the formation of an antigenic complex that acts as an essential guide for T cell responses. Thus, MHC restriction offers the specific immune cell the opportunity to efficiently 'see' and respond to original extrinsic antigens. In general terms, peripheral $CD8^+$ T cells recognize (via their TCR) the 'processed' antigen peptide coupled with the self MHC class I molecule, whilst the $CD4^+$ T cell 'sees' the peptide in association with MHC class II antigens. APCs which process foreign proteins, express on their cell membrane 'processed' peptide coupled with their intrinsic MHC class II antigen. That complex interacts with the $CD4^+$ T cell expressing the appropriate TCR (CD3/Ti) specific for the complex (see Fig. 1.11). The above explanation of the role of MHC molecules has received strong support from recent experiments where 'cloned' MHC genes have been incorporated in and expressed on cell types which do not normally function as APC for T cell responses. However, following MHC gene transfection they have been demonstrated to efficiently present peptide antigen for T

cell responses. Thus MHC molecules, by influencing T cell responses (the central event of most immune reactions), can be seen as important regulators of immune responsiveness.

2. The polymorphism in the MHC is seen, in evolutionary terms, as a safeguard to allow for the continuing opportunity within the species to generate responses against potentially any antigen. Additionally, with a particularly lethal antigen (e.g., a pandemic virus infection), some individuals of the species will have the required polymorphic form of the MHC to allow survival.

3. The phenomenon of immune response genes discussed previously (Section 1.2.4) has been partly explained by and demonstrated experimentally to be directly linked to MHC gene products, in some situations. Thus animals, of a particular MHC type that will not respond to certain antigens, become responders when cloned MHC genes from responder types have been introduced directly into their genome. In these situations the autosomal dominant immune response gene effect is associated with a MHC restriction element; the product of the immune response gene is in reality the appropriate MHC molecule.

Currently, other physiological roles of the MHC are being investigated, e.g., their possible involvement in very primitive cell to cell interactions, in particular with regard to pathological processes such as cancer metastases.

Non-physiological role of MHC

1. The MHC encoded class I and class II molecules have been clearly defined as the major triggers and targets in alloimmune responses associated with transplantation. *In vitro* immunological assays which particularly define the MHC effects include the mixed lymphocyte reaction (MLR), cell-mediated lympholysis (CML) assay, and other lymphocytotoxic assays including the cross-match assay (see Chapters 2 and 9).

2. MHC and disease associations. Population and family studies, using serological and cellular typing assays and, more recently, MHC gene DNA analyses (RFLP and DNA probe hybridization), have clearly revealed particular disease associations with various MHC alleles and their products. The associations occur at frequencies much higher than can be accounted for by random association. Although most disease associations have been demonstrated with MHC class II molecules, the two strongest associations, quantified as relative risks (RR), are seen with MHC class I molecules (HLA-B27) and ankylosing spondylitis (AS) and Reiter's syndrome. Table 1.3 gives some examples of well-established HLA antigen repertoire and certain diseases.

There are some interesting general features which characterize many HLA disease associations:

Table 1.3. HLA associations and disease

HLA type			
Class I	**Class II**	**Disease**	**Approximate relative risk (RR)**[a]
	DR2	Narcolepsy[a]	>300
B27	–	Ankylosing spondylitis	~90
B27	–	Reither's syndrome	~40
	DR3	Insulin-dependent Diabetes mellitus	~5
	DR4		~5
	DR3/4		20
	DR4	Rheumatoid arthritis	~5
	DR4	IgA nephropathy	~4
	DR2	Pemphigus vulgaris	24
	DR3/DR7	Coeliac disease	~10
	DR3	Systemic lupus erythematosus	~4
		Grave's disease	~3

[a] The relative risk (RR) is a statement of the chance an individual, with the disease-associated HLA antigen, has of developing the disease compared with an individual who lacks that HLA type. The higher the RR the more frequent is that antigen represented in the patient population.
[b] In excess of 99 per cent of narcolepsy patients are reported to be HLA-DR2 but larger studies are needed for absolute confirmation of this association.

1. The diseases are often of unknown aetiology and pathophysiology.
2. There is a hereditary pattern with weak penetrance.
3. Many of the diseases have associated immune abnormalities, with features of autoimmunity.
4. Environmental factors—special microbial antigens are suspected as being part of a multifactorial aetiopathology.

Population studies allow a statistically significant association between a particular HLA gene product and a disease to be established, but they neither reveal the mechanism involved nor provide definitive evidence of genetic linkage between putative disease susceptible gene(s) and the MHC gene. In contrast, family studies can reveal such genetic linkage. Some of the traditional mechanisms put forward to explain the HLA disease associations can be summarized as follows.

There may be *molecular mimicry*, especially with respect to 'complementarity' between a pathogen and an HLA molecule or a closely linked gene product. As a result, the immune system is unable to discriminate between 'self' (i.e., HLA antigen) and a 'non-self' pathogen, with a resultant failure to eliminate/inactivate the pathogen. Some experimental evidence supports (albeit weakly) such a hypothesis for the association of B27 with ankylosing spondylitis and possible Gram-negative bacteria, the latter possessing glycoprotein conformations similar to B27.

The association may be due to HLA molecules in susceptible individuals acting as receptor molecules for potential pathogens. This suggestion implies that at the protein or nucleic acid level one would expect to find subtle differences (e.g., in the HLA-DR3 molecule) between a patient with the disease and a normal individual who also possesses DR3.

The MHC genes may be closely linked to immune response (IR) genes, which can be dominant or recessive, and whose presence or absence will determine the magnitude of response (or lack of it) to environmental antigens which may contribute toward the disease process. In fact, experimental studies in animals of well-defined inbred strains have produced evidence for the existence of IR genes, and that some of the animal class II MHC genes actually function as IR genes. Recently, more limited evidence in humans has indicated that some D region molecules may represent examples of human IR genes.

1.3.2 B lymphocytes, receptors, and antibodies

Mature B lymphocytes express as an integral part of their membranes, immunoglobulin glycoproteins which function as the specific antigen receptors. These B cells, following antigen binding to the receptor and appropriate activation, can proliferate and differentiate into immunoglobulin producing and secreting plasma cells. Some B cells fail to reach the end stage of plasma cell development, but after mitotic division may revert to surface membrane immunoglobulin (smIg) receptor-bearing *memory B cells*. The basic structure of the immunoglobulin receptor is shown in Fig. 1.9. This is also the structure of secreted immunoglobulin found in blood and other body secretions. Immunoglobulin molecules of known antigen-binding specificity are called antibodies. The terms are often used synonymously.

Plasma cells produce and secrete all classes and subclasses of antibodies: IgM; IgG(1–4); IgA(1–2); IgD; and IgE. The latter are associated with either kappa (κ) or lambda (λ) light chains on individual molecules. Single heavy chains of immunoglobulin are never found with mixed κ and λ chains. Table 1.4 summarizes some definitions and properties of immunoglobulin-antibody molecules. In their development from the lymphoid stem cell, the earliest B lineage cells do not have antibody receptors on their membrane, but can be defined by the presence of other differentiation molecules, such as CD19 (see Section 1.2.1). The cell designated the pre-B cell has restricted to its cytoplasm the heavy chain (μ) of IgM with no associated light chain. Figure 1.5 shows the sequences in the normal development of the B cell, with some of the important markers recognized on the cells, and some of the genetic events occurring during this development.

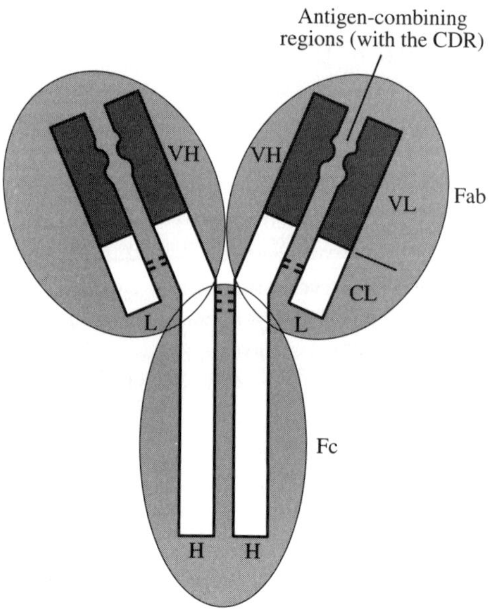

Fig. 1.9. Basic structure of an immunoglobulin-antibody molecule and the surface immunoglobulin antigen receptor on B lymphocytes. CDR, complementary determining regions; Fab, fragment antigen binding domain; Fc, fragment crystallizable domain; H, heavy chain; L, light chain; V, variable region; C, constant region.

B cells are produced continuously in human bone marrow throughout life and it is estimated that more than 10^8 cells are formed every day. It is calculated that such production provides in excess of 10^6 clones of B cells (each clone expressing an antibody receptor with a unique antigen specificity—clonal selection theory), ample provision for the diversity of human antibodies necessary to counteract the potential universe of antigens.

The immunogenetics of immunoglobulin (receptor and secreted antibody) production provides evidence to support the clonal selection theory and to explain specificity and diversity. The genes for immunoglobulin heavy chains are found on chromosome 14 whilst the genes for κ and λ light chains are found on chromosomes 2 and 22 respectively. In all nucleated cells these genes can be demonstrated to be in what is termed a '*germ line*' configuration. In a given cell only the maternal or paternal genes are selected for expression (not both) by a process termed *allelic exclusion*.

The term 'gene' applies to discontinuous segments (sequences) of nucleotide bases. The stretches of bases containing the information that will be transcribed to mRNA and translated to immunoglobulin-antibody

Table 1.4. Some definitions and properties of antibodies

Definitions

1. *Basic antibody unit*: (see Fig. 1.9.) Heavy chain – pair of high molecular weight chains – defines the classes of antibody.
2. *V and C regions*: V (variable) regions contain marked variability of amino acid sequences between different antibody molecules; C (constant) regions contain very little variability
3. *Antigen-binding sites*: formed by small numbers of amino acids in the V regions of heavy (H) and light (L) chains.
4. *Antibody classes*: 5 classes of immunoglobulins in man – IgG, IgM, IgA, IgD, and IgE – defined by determinants in the H chains which are respectively denoted as γ, μ, α, δ, ϵ. Subclasses are found in the IgG and IgA immunoglobulins.
5. *Polymer forms of antibodies*: composed of more than one of the basic monomer units. Thus, IgM in blood is usually pentameric (5 basic units link by disulphide bridges). IgA occurs as a dimer in body secretions, linked by disulphide bonds together with an additional polypeptide called secretory component.
6. *Genes encoding* H chain V regions are VDJ and encoding L chain V region are V and J. C genes encode the corresponding H and L chain constant regions.

Properties

	IgG	*IgM*	*IgA*	*IgD*	*IgE*
Heavy chain	γ	μ	α	δ	ϵ
Subclass chains	γ_1, γ_2, γ_3, γ_4	–	α_1, α_2	–	–
L chain	κ or λ	κ or λ	κ or λ	κ or λ	κ or λ
Mol. weight	150 000	900 000	160 000 monomer 400 000 dimer	180 000	190 000
Serum half-life	28 days	4–5 days	4–5 days	2–8 days	1–5 days
Complement fixation	++	+++	±	–	–
Placental transfer via Fc region	yes	no	no	no	no
Binding to mast cells via Fc region	γ_4 (?)	no	no	no	+++
Anti-bacterial	+	+++	+	±	±
Anti-viral	+	++	+++	–	–
Fc binding to phagocytes	+++	±	+	–	+ (eosinophils and macrophages)

protein are termed *exons* and the intervening non-encoding sequences are termed introns. The exons encoding for different parts of the antibody molecule are named V, D, J, and C for the heavy chains, and V, J, and C for the light chains. The critical point to note is that cells which are committed along the pathway of B lymphoid development change their germ line configuration of the immunoglobulin 'gene' elements (the V, D, J, C exons) by undergoing so-called *somatic rearrangement*—bringing together the gene exons by the removal of the intervening introns. The rearrangement process involves various nuclear enzyme systems and subtle nucleic acid curling, splicing, and recombining events. The end result is the product of a final mRNA transcript which is translated into an immunoglobulin protein. In pre-B cells only the IgM—V, D, J, C—genes are rearranged and expressed as μ heavy chain protein in the cytoplasm. In the immature B cell the μ gene element is present along with genes for V, J, and C for either κ or λ. Mature B cells rearrange and express IgM and IgD heavy chain genes, both of which are associated with the same rearranged light chain on the cell membrane. Thus, the antigen receptor on mature B cells is composed of IgM and IgD, but both Igs use the same light chain for association and have the same antigen binding specificity, i.e., the same V region (see Fig. 1.9).

At the gene level there are many alternative V, D, and J gene segments which can combine in various combinations during rearrangement, and can then be translated into many alternative V-region proteins for both heavy and light chains. These numerous possible combinations of V–D, J or V–J provide the major part of the genetic basis for diversity implicit in the clonal selection theory. Each combination contributes to a novel receptor; similarly, each individual combination provides part of the unique specificity of the individual clone.

The basis of diversity and specificity can also be seen in the amino acid sequences of antibody proteins. The V regions of heavy chains show segments of extreme amino acid variability between the N termini (Fig. 1.9) of differing antibodies of the same class. Different Igs with different antigen-binding specificities show marked amino acid differences in their V regions which correspond with the points of contact and binding of antigen. These so-called '*hypervariable regions*' (3 to 4 in number) correspond to the complementarity determining regions (CDR) which interact with antigens. The term '*idiotope*' is used to define the unique sequence of amino acids associated with the unique specificity of a single hypervariable region. Antibodies recognizing and defining the unique confirmation contributed by the combination of CDRs in heavy- and light-chain V regions are called *anti-idiotypes*, i.e., the idiotype is the summation of the epitopes derived from the combination of CDRs of heavy and light chains.

Apart from their specific antigen receptors, B cells also express other important phenotypes which can be correlated with their function. Thus, the HLA class II DR molecules on B cells have been shown to function as presenters of antigen to $CD4^+$ T cells. B cells react to antigens and produce antibody, but may also present other epitopes of the antigen to T cells for their reactivity. Similarly, receptors have been defined on B cells which bind secreted products of activated T cells, i.e., some of the interleukins (see Section 1.4.1) which in turn assist in B cell differentiation and/or proliferation events leading to antibody production and secretion. Hence, a two-way co-operation between B and T lymphocytes is becoming more apparent. Some of the other molecules defined on the surface of B cells include HLA class I antigens, receptors for complement components termed CR2 and CR3.

Diverse ligands such as Gram-negative bacterial lipopolysaccharides (LPS), Nocardia extracts, viruses such as Epstein–Barr virus (EBV), T cell lymphokines, chemicals, such as phorbol esters, and antibodies directed against the B cell immunoglobulin, can all act as mitogens (stimulators) for B cells. Following the binding of these varied ligands, singly or in various combinations, triggering of membrane-associated enzyme systems (involving turnover of inositol phospholipids and Ca^{2+} ion mobilization) results in cell cycle changes in DNA and protein synthesis in B cells. These complex interactions are currently under intense investigation. Mitogens have largely been exploited in research to dissect the details of B cell physiology; knowledge of their activity has also helped to explain clinical and laboratory observations, such as the marked proliferation of B cells, lymphocytosis, lymphadenopathy, and hypergamma-globulinaemia associated with EBV infections. Most of the clinical and laboratory findings can be explained by the mitogenic effects of EBV on B cells together with T cell responses against EBV infected B cells. Furthermore, the interaction of EBV with normal cell growth controlling gene elements, e.g., the c-*myc* proto-oncogene, offers a molecular explanation for the origin of some B cell lymphomas. The translocation of the c-*myc* oncogene from chromosome 8 to the reactive regions of the immunoglobulin genes on chromosomes 14, 2, and 22, together with the mitogenic drive of EBV for B cells, result in disorders such as Burkitt's lymphoma, and other B cell non-Hodgkin's lymphomas.

The molecular rearrangements of immunoglobulin genes, together with the definition of light chains and idiotypes on the B cell antigen receptor, have been readily exploited in clinical medicine to characterize lymphoid neoplasia. The surgeon who is called on to remove lymph nodes during the clinical investigation of lymphadenopathy, may find that the B cells in the removed specimen all express one type of light chain, thus indicating a 'clonal' neoplastic proliferation. In a normal or reactive node, analysis reveals approximately 60 per cent κ and 40 per cent λ positive cells. Recently, anti-idiotypic MABs have been used in the immunotherapy of clonal B cell malignancies.

In more difficult and complex analyses, the neoplastic nature of the B cells is defined by demonstrating the presence of the predominant and most widespread idiotype. These sophisticated examples of phenotyping, when necessary, can be complemented by genotypic analysis using DNA probes to define gene rearrangement events in clonal B cell proliferation.

Primary and secondary antibody responses

Figure 1.10 shows the classic kinetics and features of the *primary* and *secondary* antibody responses following injections of an antigen. The secondary response has a shorter lag period, the antibody response is quantitatively greater and lasts longer, the quality of the antibody is better – has a stronger binding 'affinity' for the antigen, and the classes of antibody change from predominantly IgM to IgG and IgA. It is important to appreciate that, although the antibody classes (heavy chain) have changed, the antigen-binding specifity is the same (i.e., anti-X, V-region specificity is maintained). The effect of the secondary response, therefore, is to generate antibodies which will bind the antigen strongly and rapidly, and recruit effector mechanisms, such as complement and phagocytic cells, which will contribute to efficient elimination of the antigen. As discussed previously (see Clonal selection theory, p. 15), the cellular aspects of lymphocyte responses following receptor–antigen interaction, explains the basis of immunological 'memory' of the secondary antibody response. The basis of the change in antibody class is defined at the molecular level

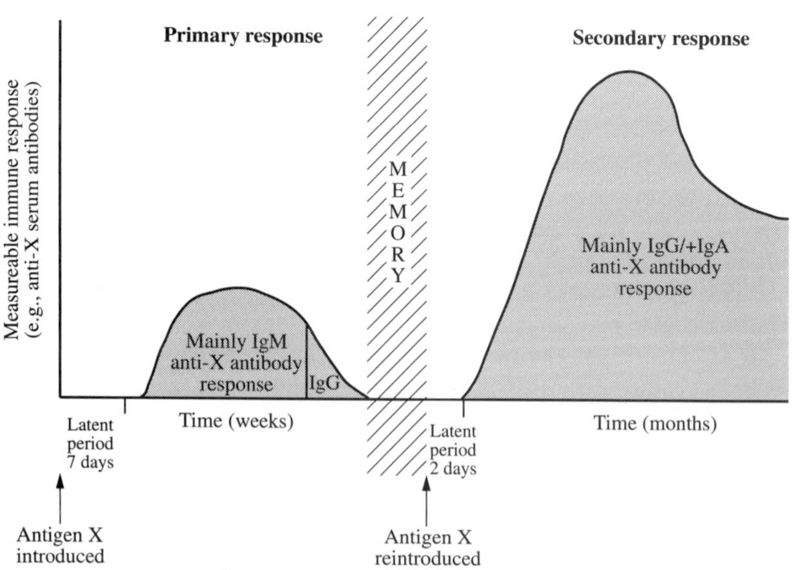

Fig. 1.10. The primary and secondary immune response.

in a so-called 'switch phenomenon'. The antibody-producing cells in the secondary response, rearrange and select IgG and IgA (γ and α C-region) rather than IgM C-region exons, whilst essentially maintaining the same V, D, J exons for the heavy chains and the V, J exons for the light chains, thus ensuring the same specificity. The molecular messages and signals responsible for isotype switching are not clear, but some evidence indicates that cell-to-cell contact between the switching B cells and certain immunoregulatory T cells is required.

1.3.3 T lymphocytes, receptors, T regulatory, and effector cells

T lymphocytes have been clearly documented as playing two outstanding roles in the immune system. They function as important *regulatory* cells and as essential *effector* cells. The most fully characterized regulatory T cell function resides within the $CD4^+$ subset and is defined as the T helper function; such cells actively assist B lymphocytes in their production of antibody. B cells and their plasma cell progeny which secrete IgG, IgA, and IgE antibodies, need a strong T helper cell contribution. Another regulatory T cell function carried out by subsets of $CD4^+$ T cells is the development and amplification of T cell cytotoxicity. The effector T cells which carry out the killing functions (e.g., of virally infected host cells) are usually located in the $CD8^+$ T cell subset; such effector $CD8^+$ T cells act most efficiently with help from the $CD4^+$ regulatory T cells. The correlation of function of cells characterized by $CD4^+$ and $CD8^+$ MABs

Table 1.5. Correlation of phenotype with effector and regulatory functions of human T cells

	Function	
	$CD4^+$ T helper/inducer	**$CD8^+$ T cytotoxic/suppressor**
Regulatory		
Help for antibody production	+	−
Help for cytotoxicity	+	−
Suppression for antibody production and CMI	−/+?	+?
Inducer of suppressor cells	+	−
Effector		
Effector cell of cytotoxicity	−	+
Effector cell of DTH	+	−

$CD4^+$ and $CD8^+$ phenotypes are recognized by the appropriate monoclonal antibodies.
These correlates are useful approximations—exceptions have been clearly documented, especially with respect to cytotoxicity and suppression (see text).

are not absolute, however, and examples have been documented where $CD4^+$ T cells have functioned as effector cytotoxic cells. Table 1.5 summarizes the main regulatory and effector function of T cells and their correlations with their CDs.

The effector roles of T cells are those of cytotoxicity, allograft rejection, and delayed type hypersensitivity (DTH). The latter describes the reaction, characterized by erythema and induration, occurring at a site approximately 24 to 48 hours following challenge with an antigen. Histologically, the lesion is characterized by an infiltrate of mononuclear cells consisting predominantly of T cells and monocytes-macrophages. Experiments have documented convincingly that $CD4^+$ and $CD8^+$ T cells are central to the development of acute allograft rejection and DTH. The term cell-mediated immunity (CMI) is used to describe those immune reactions where T cells play the predominant role (see Table 1.2), and where experimentally the reaction can be transferred passively by T cells and not by antibodies. Some examples of CMI can be summarized as follows:

- resistance to infections, especially associated with intracellular microorganisms (e.g., viruses, parasites) which display their antigens on the surface of infected cells;
- allograft rejection;
- DTH: Mantoux, lepromin test, contact hypersensitivity (e.g., with metals); and
- anti-tumour responses in man and animals (see Chapter 3).

It is clear that not all of these responses are clinically advantageous, some manifestly induce more harm (immunopathology) than benefit, e.g., DTH to industrial metals and chemicals.

T cell receptors

T cells recognize antigens specifically via the T cell antigen receptor complex (TCR) on the cell membrane. As mentioned previously, the TCR (composed of the antigen specific heterodimer, Ti, and associated closely with the CD3 molecular complex) recognizes antigen in a highly specific manner, when it is present on the cell surface in association with products of the organism's own MHC molecules. Thus, $CD4^+$ T helper cells, in most situations, see the antigen closely linked to class II MHC products (Fig. 1.11). In contrast, $CD8^+$ effector T cytotoxic cells destroy abnormal host cells which express foreign antigen or altered self antigen closely linked to class I MHC products. The distribution of MHC antigens correlates well with the 'restriction' phenomenon of T cell recognition. Class I MHC is present on essentially all cells, which can be the targets for a wide range of viral or other intracellular pathogens. Thus, via its TCR, $CD8^+$ T cells are able to recognize those cells which display the viral antigens on their surface,

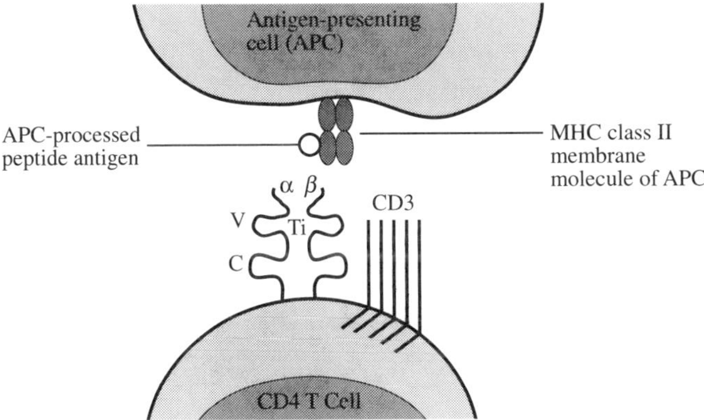

Fig. 1.11. T cell antigen-receptor unit: recognition of peptide antigen-MHC/HLA complex (MHC restriction phenomenon). CD3/Ti complex = functional T cell receptor (TCR); V, variable region; C, constant region.

usually before complete viral assembly and release. The cytotoxic T cell, therefore, is able to efficiently abrogate the infection. Experimental animal tumours, induced chemically or virally, have been shown to express 'neo-antigens' on the tumour cells which can be recognized and destroyed by T cells (see Chapter 3).

The antigen specific Ti of the TCR is a glycoprotein heterodimer molecule, comprising an α chain and a β chain which are linked by a disulphide bond in a functional receptor (see Fig. 1.11). Recent experiments, using gene transfection of isolated α and β genes, indicate that a composite conformation formed by α and β chains 'sees' the appropriate and matching conformation of the foreign antigen-MHC complex. The Ti on a $CD4^+$ T helper cell will bind to the antigen-MHC class II molecule complex on an APC. Contrastingly, the Ti on a $CD8^+$ cytotoxic T cell will bind to the antigen-MHC class I complex on the appropriate target cell. It is currently thought that the CD4 and CD8 molecules on the respective peripheral T cells play an important role in increasing the affinity of the T cell antigen recognition and binding reactions, particularly in primary T cell responses. It is envisaged that the CD4 molecule binds to non-polymorphic determinants of the MHC class II on the APC, at some distance from the antigen-MHC class II complex site. CD8 is believed to perform a similar role, enhancing the binding to comparable determinants on the MHC class I molecule.

It should be made clear that the T cell receptor (Ti) is not immunoglobulin, as is the case for the B cell antigen receptor. Nevertheless, Ti has a comparable molecular genetic arrangement whereby the separate genetic loci, designated V, D, J, and C gene segments, are found in the germ line of cells committed to a T lymphoid lineage (early in the thymus environment). The genes undergo somatic rearrangement events (similar to those described for the B cell receptor) resulting in the transcription and translation of protein 'messages' for the Ti receptor molecule, which becomes expressed on the T cell membrane closely linked with the CD3 molecule. The CD3/Ti complex (TCR) appears to be essential for proper triggering of T cells following interaction with the antigen-MHC complex. Specificity is the property of the Ti α/β heterodimer and can be shown to be associated with the V-region determinants. Diversity is due to V regions associating with different D, J, and C combinations. Like B cell receptors, idiotypic determinants can be shown to be associated with the V region of the Ti of the TCR.

Recently, a second TCR has been described with a functional receptor complex (Ti) comprising a γ (gamma) and δ (delta) heterodimer, distinct from α/β and encoded by separate genes. The precise role of this second receptor is unclear, but there are indications of its usage by some peripheral cytotoxic T cells and of a prominent role in anti-mycobacterial responses. Within the thymus it precedes the α/β receptor and may play a role in the thymic selection events associated with T cell development (see the section on the thymus, p. 10). Nevertheless, the majority of T cell receptors found on most of peripheral T cells are the classical α/β Ti, associated with CD3.

Regulatory T cells

How do T cells carry out their regulatory and effector functions? Several clear facets of regulatory action have been established. Thus, $CD4^+$ T helper cells (for B cell production of antibody) have been shown to produce *lymphokines* (soluble, small polypeptide hormones), which bind to appropriate receptors on the B cell membrane and contribute to B cell activation. Examples of such T cell lymphokines include interleukin-4, -5, and -6, and to a lesser extent interleukin-2 (see Section 1.4.1).

The regulatory T cells which amplify effector cytotoxic T cells do so largely by producing and secreting the lymphokine interleukin-2 (IL-2) which binds to the IL-2 receptor expressed on the membrane of the $CD8^+$ cytotoxic cell. Antigen-responding T cells, as part of their activation process, express on the surface of the cell membranes the classic receptor for IL-2, termed TAC or the interleukin-2 receptor (CD25). TAC represents one of several *activation molecules* expressed by responding T cells, and usually detectable on the cell membrane within 24 hours of the T cell TCR-antigen interaction. Various other activation markers appear subsequently on the proliferating T cells and include MHC-encoded HLA-DR and 'late' markers, such as the very late activation antigen-1 (VLA-1). Resting, non-activated, mature T lymphocytes do not express these activation markers.

Apart from antigen triggering of T cells (via their TCR), the cells can also be activated by mitogens such as plant-derived lectins, e.g., phytohaemagglutinin (PHA) and concanavalin A (CON A) which stimulate T cells into activation and proliferation. The lectins bind to receptors (non-TCR sugar moieties) on many different T cell clones (polyclonal) and induce mass cell activation. MABs directed against certain CD antigens of T cells can also function as mitogens for cell activation. MABs directed to epitopes of CD2 and CD3 can trigger activation, but the right monoclonal must be chosen, because others directed to different epitopes of the same CD can lead to T cell death or inactivation. In fact, one of the therapies used to suppress an intractable acute renal allograft rejection episode is an anti-CD3 MAB (termed OKT3).

Effector T cells

The lethal signal delivered by cytotoxic T cells to their target antigens (e.g., virally infected cells, or tumour cells) is not clearly defined. It requires close cell-to-cell contact and probably involves the release of toxic granules (basic proteases) from the T cell cytoplasm, which disrupt the membrane integrity of the target cells.

The effector T cells associated with the DTH reaction have been shown to mediate the local changes, predominantly by the action of a series of lymphokines. Locally released interleukin-2 attracts and leads to the activation/proliferation of many other T cells recruited into the DTH lesion, as well as increasing monocyte-macrophage activity. Another T cell lymphokine, interferon gamma (IFN-γ), also attracts and activates macrophages in sites of DTH (see Section 1.4.2). These events lead to a cascade of other factors and cell-to-cell interactions which ultimately lead to the formation of granulomas. The time required for lymphokine synthesis and secretion by T cells, following their interaction with 'antigen', accounts for the time 'delay' which is synonymous with DTH.

There is evidence, from *in vivo* and *in vitro* experiments of the phenomenon of down-regulation of both humoral and CMI responses. Previous experiments have tended to indicate that suppression is associated with and mediated by the CD8$^+$ T cell subset, both in man and in experimental animals. However, more recent studies, involving the isolation of T cell clones and identification of their functional molecules of specificity, have highlighted the difficulty of isolating and demonstrating a T cell clone which can be called a suppressor T cell. This is in contrast to the ease of isolation and demonstration of functional CD8$^+$ T effector cytotoxic clones, and CD4$^+$ T helper clones. Accordingly, there is now doubt as to whether a distinct T cell or T cell lineage exists which can be called a suppressor T cell. In transplantation studies, elegant experiments have repeatedly demonstrated that transfer of lymphoid cells from experimentally manipulated animals will suppress allograft rejection in naïve animals. So, where are the suppressor cells in the transferred lymphoid cells and why are they not clonable as $CD8^+$ T cells? The current view is that in many situations it is difficult to establish the presence of a distinct subset of T cells with suppressor function, even though functional suppression is readily and repeatedly demonstrated. However, within defined micro-environmental settings and experimental circumstances, some cells in the $CD4^+$ and $CD8^+$ populations can respond in such a manner as to result in the inhibition or suppression of immune reactivity *in vivo*. Thus, if a $CD8^+$ T cytotoxic effector cell is generated against a $CD4^+$ T cell, which is responsible for a DTH reaction, the killing of that $CD4^+$ T cell will result in the 'suppression' of the DTH immune response. Similar examples could be given for down-regulation of a B cell antibody response. Hence, cytotoxic T cells recognizing and reacting against the idiotype on a particular responding B cell clone could lead to deletion of the specific antibody response—manifesting clinically as specific humoral antibody suppression. Additionally, gene products of the MHC-D (DR, DQ) region, in particular circumstances during an immune response, may function as down-regulating or suppressing elements. More research is required for a better understanding of suppression and the factors responsible for it.

1.3.4 Antigen-presenting cells and adhesion molecules

Most antigen-processing and -presenting cells (APCs) can be defined as members of the mononuclear phagocyte series (MPS). Table 1.6 lists the location of some well known MPS cells. The latter have been shown to

Table 1.6. Location of some mononuclear phagocytes and antigen-presenting cells

Location	**Cell**
Bone marrow and blood	Monocytes and low density dendritic cells (mobile)
Tissue sites (widespread)	Macrophages (mobile)
Lymph node	Follicular dendritic cells (in B cell follicles)
	Interdigitating dendritic cells (T cell areas—paracortex)
Connective tissue	Histiocytes (mainly sessile)
Skin	
Epidermis	Langerhans cells (LC)
Dermal	Indeterminate cells (CD1 positive)—LC precursors
Liver	Küpffer cells (fixed)
Bone	Osteoclasts
Nervous system	Microglial cells
Spleen lymph node, bone marrow	Macrophages (fixed)
Serous cavities	Peritoneal and pleural macrophages

be derived from pluripotential stem cell precursors committed to the generation of monocytes-macrophages. Partially committed stem cells for the MPS, in *in vitro* culture, give rise to mixed colonies of granulocytes and macrophages. MPS-committed stem cells have been shown to be completely different from lymphoid stem cell precursors.

The maturation and proliferation of MPS cells is partly controlled by specific growth factors, called colony-stimulating factors (CSFs), some of which are produced by fibroblasts and lymphocytes. Among the well-defined glycoprotein CSFs known to affect MPS of cells are the granulocyte-macrophage CSF (GM-CSF) and the monocyte CSF (M-CSF). Other secreted polypeptides from leucocytes also induce MPS cell activation-differentiation and proliferation, and includes interleukin-3, which has multiple-CSF activity.

Previously, the CSFs were obtained from crude cell supernatants and extracts and their properties defined by intricate biological assays. The recent availability of pure recombinant DNA-derived CSFs have played a significant part in clarifying the role of the various CSFs, and has resulted in studies evaluating their use in clinical practice. In clinical situations of marrow hypofunction or aplasia, such as following chemotherapy, radiotherapy or in aplastic anaemia, or the intractable anaemia associated with chronic renal failure—clinical trials have already commenced using defined CSFs to stimulate normal haemopoeisis.

The MPS cells play varying roles in the early (afferent) events of immune reactions as well as in the final effector (efferent) responses of humoral and CMI. Their role in the afferent response relates mainly to their ability to process and appropriately present antigens to the lymphocytes with the specific receptors for the antigenic epitopes. MPS cells have varying abilities as antigen-presenting cells (APCs). Langerhans cells in the skin, dendritic cells in the B cell follicles of lymph nodes, interdigitating dendritic cells in the T cell paracortical areas of nodes, and low density circulating dendritic cells in the blood and lymph ('veiled' cells) are known to be excellent APCs. On a cell-to-cell basis, the latter are more efficient APCs than circulating monocytes and tissue macrophages. The characteristic properties of these APCs are their abilities for limited phagocytosis and controlled partial degradation of antigens, and the subsequent re-expression of the antigenic fragments associated with the endogenous/constitutive MHC class II molecules of the APC. The relevance of controlled antigen processing and presentation can be appreciated by considering granulocytes, which express MHC class II antigens and can phagocytose antigens extremely well. Nevertheless, granulocytes are extremely poor APCs. Once inside their cytoplasmic phagosomes, the antigen is soon exposed to a devastating array of lysosomal enzymes following fusion of the phagosome with the lysosome. The antigen is then almost completely degraded, with no useful fragments remaining for presentation.

The fine details of how APCs control the degradation of protein antigens to immunogenic peptides and the sites in and on the APC where the peptides associate/complex with the MHC molecules is currently under intense investigation. There is evidence that intracellularly generated peptides may be associated within cytoplasmic endosomes with newly synthesized MHC molecules, the complex then being expressed on the cell membrane. Apart from efficient presentation of antigen fragments, APCs also secrete the soluble factor *interleukin-1*, which sends accessory signals to the T cell to aid its activation.

'Adhesion' molecules

These molecules are involved in the adherence to and intimate contact of granulocytes and other inflammatory cells to vascular endothelium, a prerequisite for the extravascular migration of cells to sites of inflammation. These molecules play a fundamental role in cell-to-cell interactions and thereby in maintaining tissue integrity. Their expression (or lack of it) on malignant cells is being investigated with regard to cancer metastases. The main adhesion glycoproteins, which have been grouped into the CD11 classification (see Section 1.2.1.) have been defined and are named LFA1, CR3, and p150, 95. The molecules are made up of two chains, the α chains being designated CD11a, CD11b, and CD11c respectively, but they share a common β chain—CD18. Patients have been described who have deficiencies of these glycoprotein adhesion molecules; not surprisingly,

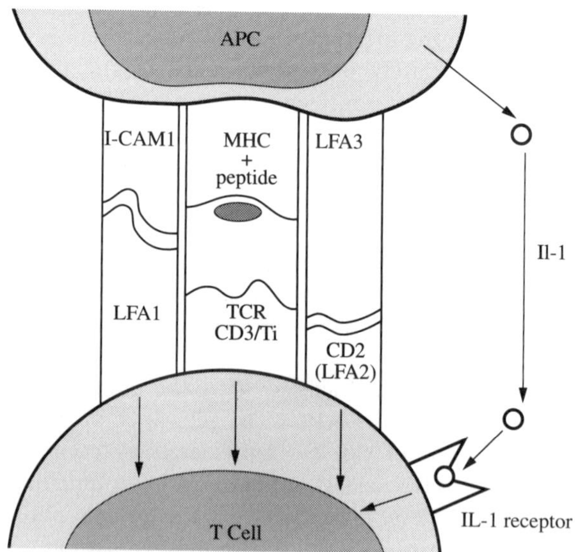

Fig. 1.12. Role of 'adhesion' molecule interactions in T cell responses to antigen present on antigen-presenting cells (APC). IL-1, interleukin → positive signals for T cell 'activation'.

they have been shown to suffer from recurrent infections and on occasions to die from their inability to mount protective inflammatory responses.

Lymphocyte function antigen 3 (LFA3), is a widely distributed cell surface glycoprotein which has been demonstrated to bind strongly to the CD2 molecule on T cells (Fig. 1.12). The CD2 molecule is sometimes referred to as LFA2. Thus, the initiation of a T and B lymphocyte response against original protein antigen is substantially enhanced by interaction with the adhesion molecules. Clearly, the intimate contact of the three main immune cell types (T, B, and APC) is important for the initiation of the full immune response. Figure 1.12 illustrates the proposed role of the LFA adhesion molecules in the interaction of the APC with the T lymphocyte. Specific recognition of the *MHC-antigenic peptide* complex is by the T cell receptor (TCR). The CD2 molecule on the T cell binds strongly the LFA3 molecule expressed on the APC, whilst the LFA1 molecule binds primarily to a widely distributed protein termed intercellular cell adhesion molecule (I-CAM) of which two forms have been recently described (I-CAM1 and I-CAM2). The adhesion molecule interactions contribute to the release of strong accessory signals for T cell activation.

Overview of interacting cells and molecules in the initiation of the immune response

In this overview major elements of the immune response are summarized. Consider a foreign non-self substance, antigen X, entering the body via natural portals of entry, or as a result of medical or surgical intervention. The complex antigen X may possess native conformational antigenic determinants which will be recognized by B lymphocytes with the appropriate antibody receptors of IgM/IgD on their cell membranes. The same antigen may also possess 'hidden' determinants, which are first exposed by processing within APC, and are subsequently expressed as small peptides on the cell membrane of the APC associated with the MHC class II molecules of the same cell. The antigen-derived peptide-MHC complex is then recognized and interacts with the appropriate T cell and its receptor. The APCs are found in strategic sites and are closely juxtaposed to T and B lymphocytes. Familiar APCs are tissue macrophages-histiocytes, blood monocytes, and related circulating low density dendritic cells, Langerhans cells of skin, and related dendritic cells of lymphoreticular tissues. Modified APCs are also found in the aggregates of lymphoid tissues associated with mucosal sites. Thus 'M' cells, which are modified macrophages/APCs, are found in the epithelium overlying Peyer's patches in the alimentary tract, and dendritic cells are found in tonsillar lymphoid tissue and in the lymphoid collections in the respiratory and urogenital tracts. In all the locations described, the APCs have the opportunity of close contact with resident T and B lymphocytes and with the pool of recirculating cells. Ample opportunities occur for the clones of T and B lymphocytes, with their respective antigen receptors, to encounter and be selected for responses, by antigens associated with the APCs. The APCs and responding T and B lymphocytes are brought into close proximity by the various adhesion molecules thus facilitating the activation and triggering of the immune response.

1.4 Connecting soluble elements of immune reactions

It is clear that in the generation of an efficient immune response there is a requirement for close cell-to-cell contact and the concomitant action of soluble, short-acting, secreted cell products. The nomenclature for these soluble elements has still to be precisely defined. Nevertheless, certain terms are in common usage and have general acceptance.

Cytokines is the term applied to a soluble factor secreted by a cell that can be shown to affect and regulate the function of that (autocrine) or other cells (paracrine). Cytokines produced by and released from lymphocytes are termed lymphokines and those from monocytes-macrophages are referred to as monokines. Originally, many of the cytokines were characterized by complex biological assays and using crude cell supernatants. As a result, various descriptive names, such as migration inhibition factor, were used to describe these functionally active molecules. By using biochemical purification techniques, and latterly gene cloning (recombinant DNA technology), many cytokines have been well characterized and are now available as pure products—*interleukins*. The latter are involved not only with white cell interactions but also can be shown to have a wide range of effects on non-lymphoreticular cells.

Several general points concerning cytokines should be appreciated:

1. They have no 'specificity' for binding antigen, as is present in the T and B lymphocyte receptors, and in the antibody V regions.
2. They are small polypeptides with short 'half-lives' in serum.
3. The target cells to which they bind usually express specific receptor molecules, some with documented ligand-receptor kinetics.
4. The binding of the cytokines to the cell membrane receptor commonly leads to DNA/RNA synthesis, and phenotypic and functional changes in the cell. Hence, cytokines regulate and modulate immune responses and inflammation, by affecting activation, proliferation, and effector functions of cells.

An outline of the main interleukins and other important cytokines closely associated with immunological reactions is given below.

1.4.1 Interleukins

Interleukin-1 (IL-1)

This refers to two closely related polypeptides (~17 kDa) termed IL-1α and IL-1β (encoded by separate genes) which appear to compete for the same receptor, and to qualitatively subserve similar functions. The following comments refer to these molecules collectively as IL-1. Originally, this interleukin was shown to be produced and secreted by macrophages-monocytes and other APCs and to play a crucial role in T cell activation. IL-1 is essential for T cell proliferation as it causes the induction/synthesis of IL-2 and the expression of IL-2 receptor by antigen or mitogen-activated T cells (see Section 1.3.3). Thus APCs 'present' antigen to T cells as well as secrete IL-1 which enhances T cell activation and proliferation.

Experiments with recombinant DNA-derived IL-1 have confirmed that this cytokine has a wide range of effects on many cell types and organs not associated with the immune system. Furthermore, a wide range of cells apart from macrophages are now known to secrete IL-1 (see Table 1.7) indicating the inappropriateness of the nomenclature. IL-1 affects, to a varying degree, the activation, proliferation, cytokine synthesis/secretion, and catabolism of a wide range of cell types including granulocytes, chondrocytes, osteoblasts, mesangial cells, fibroblasts, and skeletal muscle cells, to name but a few. This apparent pleiotropic effect of IL-1 is best considered as part of an adaptive, broad-based (non-specific), evolutionary response to noxious stimuli and tissue damage. This results in the induction of mechanisms which may lead to the destruction and elimination of

Table 1.7. Some biological consequences of interleukin-1 on various cell types

T cell: activation/proliferation of CD4 and CD8 T cells	
B cell: growth and differentation	Many of these activities contribute to a broad-based inflammatory/ acute phase response
Hepatocytes: acute phase protein release	
Chondrocytes: release of enzymes	
Endothelial cells: increased proliferation	
Hypothalamus/thalamus: induction of fever and somnolence	
Granulocytes: mobilization from bone marrow and chemo-attraction to site of inflammation	
Muscles	
Fibrous elements	
Cell sources of IL-1: Macrophage-monocytes, keratinocytes, astrocytes, Langerhans cells, large granular lymphocytes, endothelial cells, renal mesangial cells	

pathogens, as well as the enhancement of repair processes within the organism—'*acute phase response*'. A wide variety of microbial products, including bacterial lipopolysaccharides, induce the production of IL-1 from macrophages. The fever induced by 'endogenous pyrogens' following infections is largely due to this enhanced production of IL-1 which has been shown to bind to receptors in the hypothalamic region and to effect thermoregulation. IL-1 activity on skeletal muscle causes proteolysis and results, in part, in the clinically observed 'wasting' associated with severe and protracted infections. Such ubiquitous activity, if associated with maladaptive, excessive or continuous production and secretion of IL-1, can contribute to the development of pathological lesions. The prolonged activity of IL-1 on chondrocytes is believed to contribute significantly to cartilage matrix damage in lesions of rheumatoid arthritis (RA), where activated macrophages and lymphocytes abound. Indeed, synovial fluid from the joints of RA patients contains increased levels of IL-1, and experimental injection of IL-1 into the joints of animals has reproduced some aspects of the pathological lesions seen in humans.

A potent source of IL-1 release is injured tissue. In surgery, some of the clinical effects seen after trauma and sepsis are in part a consequence of the action of enhanced levels of circulating IL-1. These include neutrophil leucocytosis, pyrexia, arthralgia/myalgia, muscle weakness and wasting (also of subcutaneous tissue), and weight loss. There are also increased plasma levels of acute phase reactants (e.g., C-reactive protein, clotting factors) due to the action of IL-1 on hepatic metabolism, with concomitant reduction in the levels of albumin, pre-albumin and transferrin (see Chapters 4 and 5 for further details).

Currently, there is intense research being carried out into developing IL-1 inhibitors which may have clinical usefulness. Interestingly, but not surprisingly, amongst the many documented activities of aspirin, like other non-steroidal anti-inflammatory drugs and steroids, is their partial inhibition of IL-1 production.

Interleukin-2 (IL-2)

This polypeptide (~15–17 kDa), produced almost exclusively by 'activated' T cells, has a much more restricted range of activity when compared with IL-1, which helps in its induction. IL-2's main effect is to stimulate the proliferation of activated IL-2 receptor (R) expressing T cells. IL-2 is also involved in activating the proliferation and differentiation of 'natural killer' (NK) cells and the so-called lymphokine-activated killer (LAK) cell. More recently, signals for B lymphocyte growth and increased macrophage cytotoxicity have been shown to be mediated by IL-2. Indeed, low-density (compared with activated T cell) IL-2Rs have been demonstrated on B cells and 'activated' macrophages.

The overall effect of IL-2 is to enhance the immune response to antigens. The specific cytotoxic ability of $CD8^+$ T cells against 'infected' cells and against tumour cells is increased, as is the non-specific cytotoxicity of NK and LAK cells. IL-2 induces the differentiation of NK cells and their precursors into LAK cells, thereby increasing substantially the range of target cells susceptible to such non-specific killing. IL-2 also indirectly assists the antibody response to antigen by enhancing activated T helper cell function. The classical receptor for IL-2 is the 55 kDa protein called TAC and designated CD25 – it is the low affinity binding receptor. Another intermediate affinity receptor (~75 kDa) has been recently characterized, and is constitutively expressed on NK cells. Interaction of the low affinity receptor with IL-2 results in the subsequent expression of a high affinity receptor which is a composite of the interaction of both (55 kDa and 75 kDa) receptors.

Within pathological situations, depressed synthesis of IL-2 has been defined as one of the contributory factors in the development of AIDS. Furthermore, the persistence of certain parasitic infestations appears to be due, in part, to their efficacy in suppressing IL-2 synthesis, e.g., in some forms of malaria and trypanosomiasis. Interestingly, Cyclosporin A, one of the most useful immunosuppressants in clinical practice, has been shown *in vitro* to be a potent inhibitor of IL-2 synthesis, and to a much lesser extent to affect adversely IL-2 receptor expression.

As will be discussed in Chapter 7, recombinant DNA-derived IL-2 is being used in various forms of cancer immunotherapy, exploiting its immune and non-MHC restricted cytotoxicity enhancing properties. The clinical use of large, non-physiological doses of IL-2 has demonstrated effects on various cells not associated with the immune system – induction of eosinophilia, changes in vascular endothelial cells. The latter effect ('leaky capillaries') often results in deleterious clinical side-effects.

Studies of the IL-2R (CD25) are usually directed to its membrane expression. More recently, studies have been performed, using techniques such as ELISA and RIA, to measure 'released' free CD25 levels in blood and other body fluids. These early reports have shown IL-2R levels to be useful clinical predictors of disease activity in autoimmune disorders, such as rheumatoid arthritis and systemic lupus erythematosus. Furthermore, preliminary reports have appeared indicating that the measurement of 'free' IL-2R is an excellent predictor of acute graft rejection. These early reports will require confirmation by larger and more in-depth studies.

Interleukin-3 (IL-3)

Cytokines, which affect clonal proliferation of haematopoietic progenitor cells, are collectively called colony-stimulating factors (CSFs). They are specifically identified according to the cell types which they induce to proliferate and differentiate (see Section 1.3.4) – macrophages (M-CSF), red blood cells (erythropoeitin), granulocytes, and monocytes (GM-CSF).

A cytokine noted to stimulate neutrophils, eosinophils, monocytes, megakaryocytes, mast cells, and erythrocyte precursors, was originally and not surprisingly called Multi-CSF. Recently, the gene for this cytokine has been cloned, and its product is now termed interleukin-3 (IL-3).

IL-3 has been shown to be produced mainly by activated $CD4^+$ T lymphocytes, its synthesis and secretion occurring 12 to 20 hours following activation. Hence, T cells may, via IL-3, significantly affect the growth and differentiation of early haematopoietic and lymphoid progenitor cells. Many of the effects of IL-3 have been documented by *in vitro* experiments, and its exact *in vivo* role as a pluripotent-CSF is unclear. Animal experiments have indicated that IL-3 synergizes with GM-CSF in accelerating heamatopoeitic recovery following severe myelosuppressive therapy. Thus, a potential clinical use of IL-3, alone or in combination with GM-CSF, is to hasten red cell, granulocyte, and most importantly, platelet recovery in situations of severe marrow suppression. Availability of large quantities of recombinant IL-3 and GM-CSF recently, makes such therapy possible. Consideration is also being given to exploiting the differentiation-inducing activity of cytokines as a means of cancer therapy, such that neoplastic clones with uncontrolled proliferative properties may be channelled toward cell differentiation with minimal proliferating ability.

Interleukin-4 (IL-4)

IL-4 is a T cell-derived lymphokine that has a major role in the activation and proliferation of B cells. It also stimulates, in an autocrine fashion, subsets of the T helper lymphocytes. Now that pure, recombinant forms of IL-4 are available, detailed *in vitro* experiments are documenting a wider and more complex range of activities. Recombinant IL-4 has been shown to synergize with other cytokines and to show a 'multi-CSF' type of function affecting erythroid, granulocytic, megakaryocytic, mast cell, and lymphoid lineages. Again, how relevant these observations are to the *in vivo* situation is uncertain.

IL-4 appears to be very important for the induction of certain immunoglobulin isotypes, especially IgE and IgG1. This area is currently under investigation, with the hope of identifying possible new avenues for controlling regulatory T cell subsets or B cell types which may be involved in the 'allergic' (type I hypersensitivity) response (Section 1.7).

Interleukin-5 (IL-5)

This T cell-derived lymphokine has been shown in man to induce eosinophilia, for so long recognized as an accompaniment of 'allergic' (type I) reactions, and of parasitic infections. The role of IL-5 in normal eosinophil physiology and in abnormal pathophysiologies, such as hypereosinophilic syndromes and associated cardiomyopathies, is currently under investigation.

In vitro experiments, using recombinant-derived IL-5 singly and in combination with other interleukins, are showing some selective effects on B cell and immunoglobulin isotype production.

Interleukin-6 (IL-6)

This is another T cell-derived lymphokine, whose main effect appears to be on the late phase of B lymphocyte differentiation to plasma cells. *In vitro*, it has been shown to be a potent growth factor for the neoplastic plasma cells of multiple myeloma. The role of IL-6 is being investigated in some antibody deficiency syndromes. Again, as is becoming more apparent, the use of the recombinant form of IL-6 *in vitro* clearly shows its functions to be much wider than that of an 'interleukin'. Thus, it has major differentiation-inducing effects on neuroendocrine cells and on hepatocytes. Like IL-1 it is able to induce hepatic protein synthesis and the release of acute phase proteins. It is too early to comment as to whether these documented *in vitro* effects may have any useful clinical relevance.

Interleukin-7 (IL-7)

This most recently cloned cytokine has been shown to stimulate the proliferation of very early lymphoid progenitor cells, and in particular to support the generation and proliferation of pre-B cells (Section 1.3.2).

Apart from the interleukins (1–7), there are other well-characterized cytokines which are relevant to the understanding of immunology and current scientific aspects of major disease states in surgery. These cytokines include interferon-γ and tumour necrosis factors α and β.

1.4.2 Other cytokines

Interferon (IFN)

Interferon-γ. The interferons (IFNs) were originally defined as substances that inhibited virus replication. IFN-α and- β (many different types) are produced by virus-infected cells, whereas interferon-γ (IFN-γ) is produced mainly by activated T lymphocytes, and is sometimes called 'immune'-interferon. IFN-γ, like other interferons has demonstrable anti-viral properties, but its main role is as an enhancing factor of the immune response. It can be shown to enhance the activity of NK cells and to markedly increase the activities and cytotoxic ability of macrophages. These enhancing effects contribute to controlling intracellular pathogens and enhance anti-tumour cell activities of cytotoxic T cells, NK cells, LAK cells, and macrophages.

Another well-documented effect of IFN-γ is the induction/appearance or upregulation of MHC-encoded molecules on many cell types. Cells which do not normally express the restricted MHC class II molecules (especially HLA-DR) can be induced to do so. Similarly, the MHC class I molecules expressed on cell membranes can be upregulated by IFN-γ. These effects are believed to be important in several areas of immunopathology. In autoimmune diseases, the production of IFN-γ by immune T cells infiltrating organs, such as the thyroid gland, induces MHC class II molecules on thyroid epithelial cells, which may contribute directly to the aetiopathology of autoimmune chronic thyroiditis (see Chapter 8). In patients with cancer undergoing immunotherapy the possible synergism of lymphokines, such as IFN-γ and IL-2, is being evaluated. Thus, IFN-γ may upregulate or induce the expression of tumour-associated molecules on cancer cells, which would make them more suitable for attack by IL-2 enhanced immune T and non-specific NK and LAK cells; concomitantly the IFN-γ may diminish the metastatic potential of cancer cells. Tumours which, to date, appear susceptible to these approaches include malignant melanoma, renal carcinoma, and some leukaemias (see Chapter 7).

Interferon-α (IFN-α). This cytokine has potent anti-cell proliferative and anti-tumour activity, independent of its well-known anti-viral properties. Furthermore, *in vitro* studies have shown that IFN-α markedly enhances the cytotoxic abilities of NK cells. Currently, recombinant IFN-α is the primary therapeutic agent for inducing and maintaining clinical remission in patients with Hairy cell leukaemia; it is also being evaluated as a treatment for some refractory non-Hodgkin's lymphomas, and with AIDS-associated Kaposi's sarcoma. It has unfortunately been disappointing as a therapeutic modality with a variety of solid cancers.

Tumour necrosis factor (TNF)

TNF-α (also called cachectin) is produced primarily by macrophages, whilst TNF-β (previously called lymphotoxin) is produced mainly by T lymphocytes. Both cytokines originally were shown to induce necrosis in transplanted sarcomas and cancer cell lines, *in vivo* and *in vitro*. It has now become apparent that the 'tumour necrosis' property of these molecules is of less relevance than originally thought or hoped. TNF-α and -β, although encoded by separate genes, show approximately 32 per cent homology at the DNA level and compete for the same cell surface receptor. The TNF genes are located in the MHC region on chromosome 6 in humans.

It has become clear that both of these cytokines produce many of the pleiotropic effects documented for interleukin-1. Current evidence suggests no major qualitative difference in the actions of TNF-α and -β. The major effects of TNF-α and -β can be as follows: (1) echancement of the inflammatory process; (2) modulation of the immune response; and (3) regulation of tumour growth.

(a) The inflammatory process. TNF activates the biochemical pathways for the production and release of free radicals and other lytic molecules,

and enhances the phagocytic abilities of granulocytes. Such activated cells become more efficient scavengers of microorganisms, including bacteria, fungi, and protozoa. The TNF-activated cells can be shown to increase their expression of cell adhesion molecules (I-CAM and various LFAs: Section 1.3.4). Vascular endothelium is also activated by TNF, leading to increased expression of MHC class I molecules, and procoagulant activity. TNF also induces fever in animals. These various effects of TNF, when controlled, are believed to be beneficial short-term adjuncts to the inflammatory process. It is now apparent that excess or inappropriate production of TNF can be very deleterious. TNF is now recognized to be one of the main mediators of septic shock associated with endotoxaemia. Injection of recombinant TNF into experimental animals, reproduces most of the deleterious effects associated with injection of endotoxin, including hypotension, disseminated intravascular coagulation, glomerular damage, and ultimately death. Antibody raised against TNF and passively administered to animals has been shown to protect against endotoxic shock (see Chapter 5). As implied in the original synonym for TNF-α, this molecule appears to play a major role in inducing the *cachexia* associated with chronic infection and malignant disease. Many of the deleterious effects of TNF are readily explicable by its direct action on its widespread receptor, and its induction of many other cytokines, including IL-1 and IFN-γ.

(b) Immune modulation. TNF modifies the action of T and B lymphocytes, largely due to its induction of IL-1 synthesis and release. However, TNF has also been shown to have a direct effect on the growth and differentiation of normal T and B cells, and most recently has been shown to act as an autocrine growth factor for the neoplastic B cells of chronic lymphocytic leukaemia. TNF also induces, on endothelial cells, a molecule which apparently promotes binding and egress of lymphocytes into tissues.

(c) Regulation of tumour growth. Studies with TNF have demonstrated dramatic effects *in vitro* on tumour cell lines and *in vivo* against chemically induced cancers in animals. The cytotoxic and cytostatic effects on cancer cells are both direct (leading to cell death associated with DNA fragmentation) and indirect by affecting the integrity of the vasculature of established tumours and probably by augmentation of NK cell function. However, clinical trials with TNF in patients with cancer, to date, have been disappointing. More recently, synergism of TNF and IFN-γ has been demonstrated *in vitro*, and researchers are currently investigating the use of both cytokines in cancer therapy, particularly in haematological malignancies. Some caution is required, however, for as mentioned above TNF has been shown to stimulate chronic leukaemic B cells.

Summary—interleukins and cytokines (see Fig. 1.13)

The availability of cloned cytokines is continuing to increase and clarify our knowledge about these substances. Recently, a cloned and partially characterized cytokine produced by monocytes and fibroblasts (and probably other cell types), and shown to have significant effects on neutrophil function and on T cells, has been designated interleukin-8. The ever-expanding number of cytokines (12) and their effects, documented by *in vitro* experiments, highlight the complexity of these biological modifiers and make the understanding of their biological role *in vivo* and possible applications in clinical medicine difficult to ascertain. Nevertheless, it is very likely that these molecules will be making significant contributions to clinical medicine in the very near future. The current pioneering use of cytokines, singly or in combination in the field of cancer immunotherapy, will increase our understanding of and define further clinical areas for exploitation of these fascinating molecules (see Chapter 7). Figure 1.13 summarizes some of the documented cytokine sources and cellular targets.

1.5 Interactive and augmenting elements of immunity

The primary interaction of an antibody Fab-V region with the complementary antigenic epitope can, on occasions, be sufficient to deal with the antigen, e.g., antibody neutralization of a cell-free virus. More commonly, the interacting antibody needs to recruit other cells and soluble factors to influence the final effector (secondary and tertiary) interactions which lead to antigen elimination. The two most important augmenting elements for humoral immune responses are *complement* and *phagocytic cells*. Contrastingly, cell-mediated immune responses result in effector reactions, augmented by the effects of other recruited cells, especially T lymphocytes (additional to those with the specific TCR for the exciting antigen) and macrophage-monocytes, and their secreted cytokines.

The cytokines can also augment cellular functions associated with non-MHC restricted cytotoxic cells, such as the NK and LAK cells, as well as the classical MHC-restricted $CD8^+$ cytotoxic T cells (see Section 1.4). It is apparent that the interactive elements of complement, phagocytic cells, together with NK cells are part of the phylogenetically older system of innate immunity (see Table 1.1) which synergizes with the antigen specific T and B lymphocyte adaptive immune response.

1.5.1 Complement

Invading non-self antigens such as viruses, bacteria, fungi, mismatched transfused blood cells, or organ transplants can be attacked by the complement series of blood proteins, especially if the 'antigens' have first

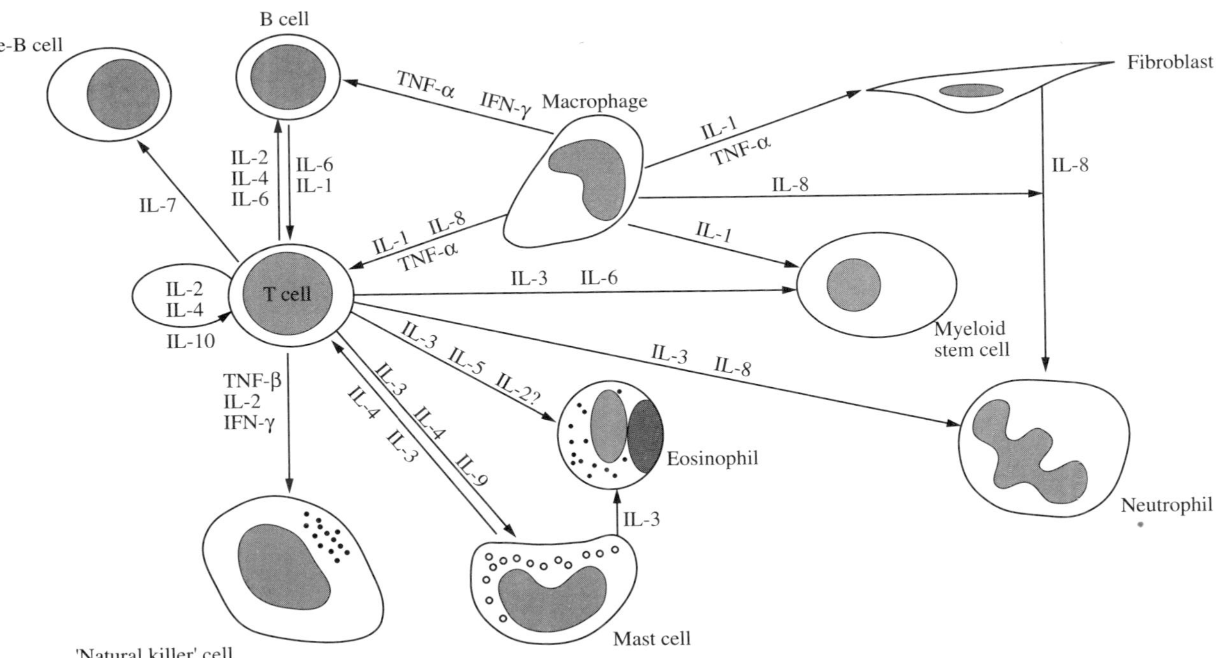

Fig. 1.13. Some cellular sources and cellular interactions of various cytokines.

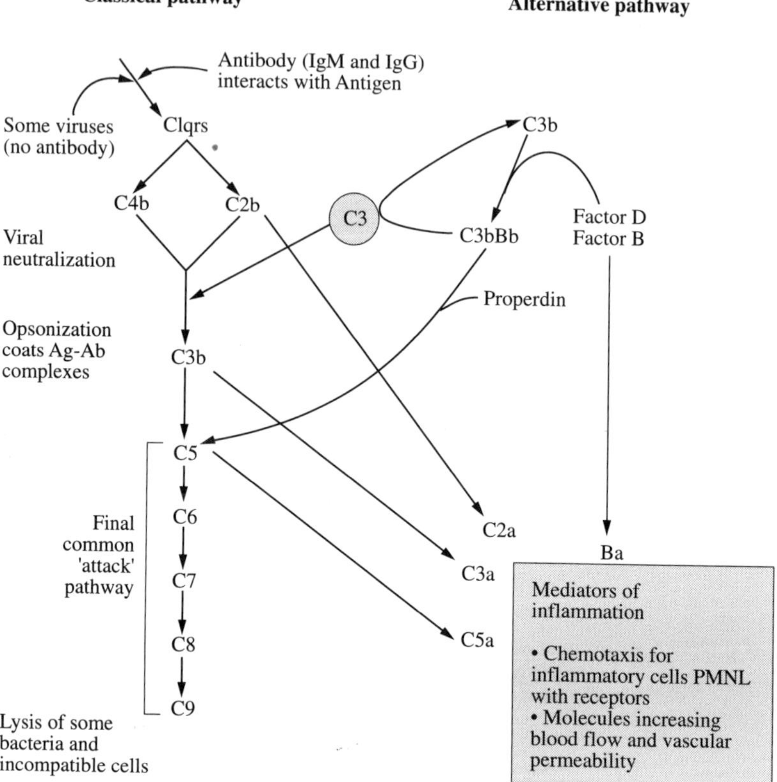

Fig. 1.14. Complement activation pathways (adapted from Chapel and Heaney 1988).

interacted with their respective antibodies. The antibody molecules on binding to the antigen undergo conformational changes, particularly associated with their Fc regions (Fig. 1.9), which makes them attractive to and provides binding sites for certain complement proteins (CIqrs) and thus leads to *complement activation* (see Fig. 1.14).

The important biological effect of activated complement is to induce and enhance inflammatory response, by increasing blood flow and vascular permeability, thus attracting granulocytes and other inflammatory cells to the site of the antibody-antigen interaction. Also it encourages leucocyte adherence to antigen and its subsequent phagocytosis. Figure 1.15 depicts the principles of opsonization associated with antibody and complement (see below). In some infections with microorganisms complement can be activated before antibody production, by intrinsic components of bacterial walls/coverings such as lipopolysaccharide endotoxins, and by the outer membrane of some viruses—this activation represents a non-specific (not antibody-directed), rapid and early defence reaction.

Activation of complement (a collective term for a series of more than 15 protein molecules found in blood, and synthesized by macrophages and related cells as well as by hepatocytes) is commonly described in terms of two pathways termed the *classical* and the *alternative* pathways. Figure 1.14 summarizes (in a simplified way) these pathways, and indicates some of the activating factors, and the useful effector responses generated by complement. The *classical pathway* is activated most efficiently by antibody-antigen complexes, particularly by IgM and IgG isotypes. C1q, the first complement component, reacts with the conformation-induced site on the antibody Fc region. The bound C1q provides attachment sites for C1r and C1s and thus generates enzyme activity (called C1 esterase) for the other components, namely C4, and then C2, which are cleaved to generate a complex termed C4b2b, which in turn acts as an enzyme to cleave the main control molecule of the complement system—C3. These early events of the classical pathway indicate the essence of the system, in which inactive precursor molecules become activated and provide attachment sites and enzymatic sites for other molecules in the series. The enzyme action produces a variety of molecules, some of which act as direct mediators of inflammation, and others provide further attachment sites for subsequent components. The complement system also has *inhibitor molecules* for the

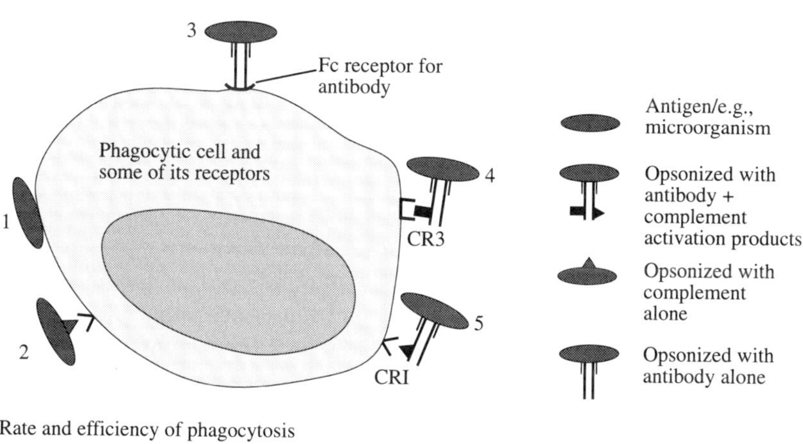

Fig. 1.15. Opsonization of microorganisms and the role of phagocytic cells, CR1, and CR3 receptors for complement activation products C3b(▲), and C3d (■).

generated enzymes, e.g., for the C1 esterase there is a C1-inhibitor molecule. The central C3 molecule is cleaved by the enzymes C4b2b, generated by the classical pathway, and C3bBb generated by the alternate pathway. These enzymes are termed C3 convertases. Other control mechanisms within the dynamic complement system include factors such as the short half-life in blood of some generated fragments, some 'decay accelerating factors', and other binding proteins. Following the action of C3 convertases, there is a final common pathway of complement activation, involving C5 to C9. The terminal activation of C8 and C9 can result in the direct lysis of some bacteria, especially Gram-negative organisms, and some susceptible cell types such as incompatible red blood cells and leucocytes. The by-products of complement activation have an important biological role *in vivo*. Thus, a key function of generated C3b is to bind to and coat antibody molecules within immune complexes. This *opsonization* of immune complexes of antibody and microorganisms (see Fig. 1.15) or antibody and soluble antigens, leads to their efficient removal and elimination from the body by cells possessing *complement receptor molecules* on their surface (termed CR1 receptors for activated C3b). CR1s are found on mononuclear phagocytes within the reticuloendothelial system and on polymorphonuclear granulocytes. Complement-derived components also play an important role in the solubilization of deposited immune complexes.

The critical role of the complement system is dramatically illustrated by rare inherited, congenital, and acquired deficiencies. Deficiencies of all the individual components and of controlling proteins have been described, and highlight some of the functions described. Patients with deficiencies of the early components of the classical pathway (Clq, r, s, C2) have tended to present with clinical features characteristic of immune complex disorders. Hence, they present with SLE-like syndromes, where the clinical manifestations are considered to be due to lack of complement-associated solubilization and removal of immune complexes, and possibly viral infections; such patients also suffer from varying degrees of recurrent infections.

Deficiency of the controlling enzyme C1-inhibitor is not uncommon and is associated with the entity angio-oedema (former name hereditary angio-neurotic oedema). Such patients commonly suffer from recurrent attacks of skin, laryngeal or intestinal oedema which may present as an 'acute abdomen'; pain and vomiting occurs with jejunal involvement and diarrhoea with colonic involvement. The acute episodes may be associated with stress or intercurrent infections. The abnormality of the C1-inhibitor can be due to a deficiency in blood or rarely to a functional defect. In the former instance, when the protein falls below a critical blood level (30 per cent of the normal), its inhibitor function on the complement system and also its inhibitor effects on plasmin and kallikrein in the coagulation pathway are compromised. Thus, C1 acts on C4 and C2 in an uncontrolled manner generating kinin-like peptides termed *anaphylotoxins*. The latter interact with receptors on tissue mast cells and vascular endothelium leading to fluid accumulation, disturbances of tissue function and activation of pain pathways. The indirect measure of C4 levels, which is nearly always abnormally low in blood, can be used as an indicator of C1-inhibitor deficiency. Treatment for C1-inhibitor deficiency and angio-oedema involves endotracheal intubation and ventilatory support in cases of life-threatening acute laryngeal oedema, avoidance of unnecessary abdominal surgery where the diagnosis is suspected from the clinical/family history, and drug treatment. Treatment with danazol, a synthetic testosterone analogue, has been shown to be effective in stimulating synthesis of functional C1-inhibitor; other therapies, including fresh frozen plasma, have been found to be beneficial. Acquired C1-inhibitor deficiency has been described in patients with various malignancies, some of whom have been shown to have a culpable autoantibody.

Patients with deficiency of C3, as a primary defect or secondary to lack of controlling inhibitors, present with severe, life-threatening recurrent bacterial infections, providing living proof of the central role of C3 in generating the critical opsonin C3b. Complement deficiencies of the late components C5–C9 have been documented. Such patients tend to present with recurrent Gram-negative septicaemia, associated arthritis or recurrent meningococcal meningitis, highlighting the essential role of complement for opsonization and lysis of these organisms.

1.5.2. Phagocytic cells

Neutrophil polymorphonuclear leucocytes (PMNLs) and macrophages-monocytes are excellent phagocytic cells which are recruited by and augment the effector reactions of the specific immune response. These cells express Fc receptors for antibody molecules (IgG, IgM), and effectively bind immune complexes as the first step in the efficient elimination of antibody-complexed antigens. The cells also have complement receptors, CR1 (for component C3b) and CR3 (for component C3d), which bind effectively to opsonized complement-coated antibody-antigen complexes for rapid and efficient clearance (see Fig. 1.15). Complement-derived fragments, such as C3a and C5a, attract PMNL by the process of chemotaxis to sites of antibody-antigen complexes, which have activated the classical pathway, and to organisms, which have activated directly the alternative pathway. PMNL degrade completely, within their phagolysosomes, the ingested antigen. Macrophages and modified phagocytic cells, on the other hand, display controlled phagocytosis with limited intracellular degradation of antigens, for subsequent expression and presentation to the appropriate antigen-specific lymphocytes (see Section 1.3.4).

The processes whereby PMNL adhere to vascular endothelium and migrate into surrounding tissues can be studied by various complex *in vitro* assays, and less efficiently by *in vivo* assays, such as the 'Reebuck' skin test. The binding to opsonized antigens, the phagocytosis and the biochemical events involved in lysosomal enzyme killing/digestion of ingested material can also be studied *in vitro*. Thus, the various energy pathways utilized by phagocytes, involving the hexose monophosphate shunt, the oxidative respiratory bursts, and the generation of superoxide and other potent radicals within the cells, are all amenable to scientific study. Such studies have indicated subtle deficiencies—genetic, congenital, and acquired—within phagocytic cells. The deficiencies range from lack of expression of molecules important for initial cell adherence interactions (Section 1.3.4) to subtle intracellular enzyme defects associated with lack of intracellular killing or antigen degradation. The common clinical feature of such phagocytic cell defects is the problem of recurrent or serious infections.

Lymphokines produced by T lymphocytes, apart from recruiting mononuclear phagocytes to sites of CMI reactions, also stimulate the phagocytic and biochemical pathways of monocytes-macrophages (see Section 1.4). Like receptors for the Fc region of antibodies and for the various components of activated complement, various receptors for cytokines, such as IFN-γ, TNF, and IL-2 are now being documented and characterized on some phagocytic cells.

1.5.3 Natural killer (NK), lymphokine activated killer (LAK), killer (K) cells

NK, LAK, and K cells will be discussed in greater detail in subsequent chapters. Some broad generalizations regarding these cell types are considered at this stage. The term NK cell describes a property which can be evaluated *in vitro* and which is believed to be operative *in vivo*. NK cells, without prior antigen sensitization, and in the absence of antibody or specific CMI, will kill a variety of cell types—autologous, allogeneic, and xenogeneic. In man, most NK cell function is found within the morphologically defined large granular lymphocyte (LGL) population. The immunophenotypic characteristics of NK cells are defined by CD16, CD56, and CD57 MABs. The classic target cell used *in vitro* to demonstrate NK cell function is K562, a primitive haemopoietic cancer cell line (see Chapter 9). The cytotoxicity associated with NK cells is non-MHC restricted, in marked contrast to the classic $CD3^+$ $CD8^+$ T cells which show class I MHC-restricted cytotoxicity.

NK cells

These cells possess various receptors for cytokines which are able to augment their killing function; receptors for IFN-γ and for IL-2 can be demonstrated on NK cells. Upon activation by the corresponding cytokines (IL-2, IFN-γ, TNF), biochemical and immunophenotypic changes (together with increased function) can be demonstrated in NK cells. *In vivo*, NK cells are assumed to be participants in the natural immune surveillance of the host against tumour cells arising due to spontaneous mutation or the action of carcinogens (see Chapter 3). Recent *in vitro* and *in vivo* experiments have demonstrated that NK cells can also have significant anti-bacterial and anti-viral effects, as well as immunoregulatory effects on developing bone marrow haematopoietic cells. The role of NK cells in allograft rejection is unclear and firm evidence is lacking in this area. A subset of NK cells can be shown to express the CD2 and CD8 molecules. However, analysis of somatic rearrangement of TCR molecules, and the use of other T cell specific CD MABs, tend to indicate that NK cells are not derived from the classic T cell lineage. Upon activation with IL-2, NK cells can be shown to develop and express the CD25 (TAC) IL-2 receptor. It is now considered that NK cells are probably the main progenitors from which lymphokine activated killer (LAK) cells are derived. The exact mode of killing of tumour/target cells by NK cells is not known. The receptor(s) on NK cells and the ligands on the target cells are imprecisely defined. Killing events are believed to be associated, in part, with the exocytosis of the characteristic granules present in NK cells and which contain many potent serine enzymes. The latter are believed to induce 'membrane lesions' leading to osmotic damage.

LAK cells

These cells show a wider range of target cell killing than NK cells, and cell lines (Daudi) which are resistant to lysis by NK cells are readily killed by LAK cells. Current evidence indicates that most LAK cells are probably derived from lymphokine (IL-2, IFN-γ)-stimulated NK cells or their progenitors. Nevertheless, it is clear that LAK activity can be associated with a more heterogeneous cell population, including a $CD3^+$ T cell which commonly lacks the CD4 or CD8 subset markers and participates in non-MHC-restricted cytotoxicity. Some authorities suggest that monocytes, with appropriate stimulation, can also exhibit LAK activity.

Currently, great efforts are being devoted to augmenting and exploiting NK and LAK activities against human tumours (see Chapter 7). *Tumour-infiltrating lymphocytes* (TIL), including LAK, MHC-restricted and other cells, isolated from surgically resected tumour specimens and expanded by lymphokine incubation *in vitro*, have demonstrated striking tumour cell killing. This cytotoxicity has been demonstrated both *in vitro* and *in vivo* and with both non-MHC and classical MHC restriction involving antigen specific cytotoxic $CD8^+$ T lymphocytes (see Chapter 2).

Killer cells

These cells, like NK and LAK cells are non-adherent, non-phagocytic mononuclear cells and are responsible for antibody-dependent cell cytotoxicity

(ADCC). In contra-distinction to NK function, these killer cells use their membrane-associated Fc receptors (for the Fc portion of an IgG antibody which has reacted with and become bound to a target cell antigen) as a bridge to approximate to and kill the antigen-bearing target cell. Apart from the classical Fc receptor-bearing, 'null' lymphocyte, a wide range of cells, including activated T cells, subpopulations of NK cells and NK precursors, as well as eosinophils and monocytes may all, under appropriate conditions, demonstrate ADCC.

1.6 Immune regulation and modulation

1.6.1. Regulatory pathways and networks

The immune system is normally an excellent self-regulatory unit. It responds to foreign, non-self antigens specifically and for a finite period, with a resultant induction of memory for the antigen, as embodied in the clonal selection theory (Section 1.2.3). An often-quoted tenet of immunology is that an efficient self-regulatory immune system does not react against self. It is now evident, however, that for the generation of an efficient and controlled immune response, a certain degree of self recognition and reaction to self components is crucial. Thus, the induction of *anti-idiotypic reactions* against the antigen-specific receptor of B and T cells, (i.e., their V domain, complementarity determining regions where antigen is bound—Section 1.3) is seen as a critical controlling factor in limiting the extent of responding B and T cell clones. At its simplest, a responding B cell receptor (smIg) or its secreted Ig (termed Antibody 1—Ab1) binds antigen and following binding, the antigen combining sites of Ab1 are conformationally altered. As a result, they in turn act as neoantigens for another B cell clone (producing Antibody 2—Ab2), this is the anti-idiotypic response (see Fig. 1.16). The *idiotype* defines the sum total of the antigenic determinants comprising the Ab1 antigen-combining sites (Fig. 1.9) and is thus highly specific for and restricted to that clone. Depending on the exactness of its fit for the antigen-combining regions of Ab1, the *anti-idiotypic antibody (Ab2)* can result in a down-regulation of the responding Ab1 clone. In some experimental systems, Ab2 (the anti-idiotype) can itself induce an anti-anti-idiotypic response (termed Antibody 3). Again with respect to exactness of fit, this Ab3 can ultimately down-regulate the Ab2 response and thus return the immune responding elements to a steady state. The Ab1 to Ab3 responses can form 'closed-loop' systems (Fig. 1.16) and hence do not go on indefinitely. The concept of anti-idiotypic responses (Ab2) is now being exploited in certain experimental systems to modulate immune responses (see below). Furthermore, in some systems, Ab3 can be shown to mimic the conformation of the exciting antigen which initially

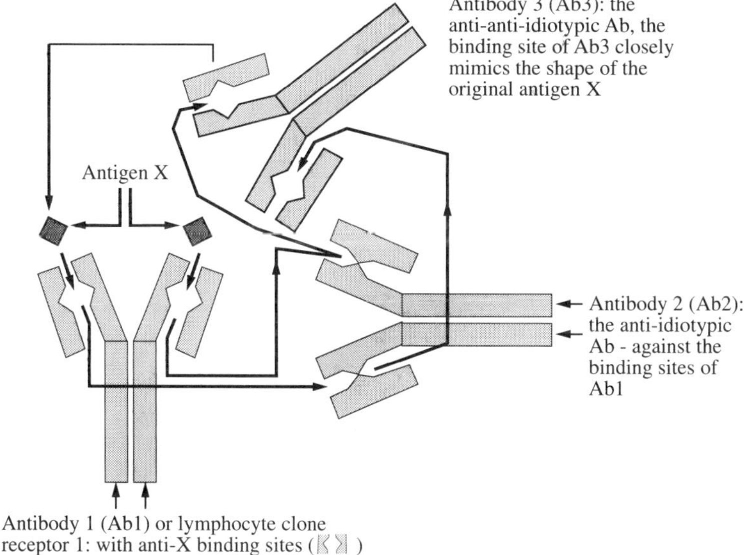

Fig. 1.16. Idiotype network responses.

reacted with Ab1. Currently, there are experimental attempts to exploit the induction of Ab3 as replacement antigens. Ab3 could replace one part of a very complex antigen (e.g., protozoal parasites), or act as an antigen to replace potentially damaging molecules or organisms (e.g., the HIV virus of AIDS) during production of vaccines. Already Ab3 antibodies have been used successfully as antigens to induce partial immunity against schistosomiasis, and as vaccination antigens to induce immunity against subsequent hepatitis B virus challenge in primates.

There is also evidence that physiological anti-self recognition may contribute to the continuous removal of effete cells. In most other situations, however, the immune system makes strenuous efforts to prevent deleterious anti-self reactions. Thus a relative tolerance to self exists. The manner of maintenance of self tolerance is classically listed as follows:

1. *Deletion of clones* expressing *high affinity* receptors with self recognition antigen-combining sites.
2. If such self reactive clones escape deletion other mechanisms exist for keeping them in a non-reacting state termed *clonal anergy*.

Recent experiments indicate that both of these mechanisms (clonal deletion and clonal anergy) operate *in vivo* to maintain the organisms state of relative tolerance to self. As detailed in Section 1.2.2, there is now convincing evidence that the thymic environment regulates, in a large part, the deletion of clones of T cells with high affinity anti-self receptors. By contrast, B lymphocytes with anti-self receptors can be isolated from the blood of individuals who are evidently not producing significant amounts of anti-self antibodies, or have no evidence of antibody-induced tissue damage. Somehow the B cell clones in question are in a state of non-reactivity (i.e., clonal anergy). The anergic state appears to be due, in part, to a lack of the necessary specific helper $CD4^+$ T lymphocytes, which are eliminated in the thymus and thus are not available to co-operate with the B cell. Most of the anti-self B cells that can be found *in vivo* (e.g., to thyroglobulin) are thus very dependent on T cell 'help'. Experimental evidence also indicates that within the peripheral lymphoid system, *immune suppressor mechanisms* may act directly in the maintenance of B cell anergy. These suppressor reactions can be clearly demonstrated experimentally *in vivo*, but with the advent of cell cloning it has proved difficult to demonstrate the existence *in vitro* of specific suppressor T or B lymphocytes. Clearly, suppression operates in normal immune regulation, but it appears not to be the property of a single cellular entity which can be characterized by a single phenotype such as a $CD8^+$ T 'suppressor cell' (see Section 1.3.3 on regulatory T lymphocytes).

3. The classic experiments of Medawar and co-workers in the 1950s and 1960s convincingly demonstrated that an immature immune system could be made tolerant to an exogenous antigen. It has long been assumed that *acquired tolerance* in T and B lymphocytes to intrinsic self antigens may also be induced during early human development. Recently, *in vitro* experiments with early developing human B lymphocytes, which express surface IgM receptors alone (in contrast to more mature B cells expressing both IgM and IgD), have demonstrated that reaction with some antigens does result in an immune paralysis of such immature B cells.

It is postulated that damaging self reactive T cell clones, which have escaped clonal deletion in the thymus, may in early ontogeny also be inactivated by contact with self antigens. An essential condition required for induction of acquired T and B cell tolerance, is that the appropriate self antigens come in contact with the specific lymphocytes during an ill-defined critical period in ontogeny. Therefore, if a self antigen is *sequestered* for anatomical reasons or undergoes changes out of phase with the developing immune lymphocytes, the opportunity for induction of acquired tolerance is lost and the potential for the development of autoimmune responses against such antigens is thus always present (see below). Which intrinsic properties of immature T and B cells render them susceptible to tolerance, rather than the induction of an immune response to antigens, are not known.

Many ingenious experimental systems suggest that antigen, antibody-antigen complexes (in various ratios), and antibody reactions with Fc receptors, may modulate immune regulatory pathways. The relevance of these various studies to the *in vivo* situation is presently unclear, and no doubt will continue to bemuse us for some time to come. What is clear, on the other hand, is that when normal regulation fails, abnormal (non-physiological) states of reaction against self become apparent in the form of autoimmune responses and autoimmune diseases.

1.6.2 Abnormal regulation and autoimmunity

A distinction should be made between autoimmune responses (with measurable autoantibodies and autoreactive T cells) and autoimmune disease where the autoreactive components can be demonstrated to play significant roles in inducing tissue and organ damage (see Chapter 8).

Autoantibodies, and to a lesser extent autoreactive T cells, can be demonstrated in a wide range of circumstances and diseases (see Table 8.1, Chapter 8). Although autoimmune disorders are heterogeneous, there are nevertheless several common features related to aetiology and pathogenesis which can be summarized as follows:

- Genetic factors.
- Immune defects.
- Hormonal factors.
- Environmental factors.

Genetic factors. Human autoimmune disorders, as well as spontaneous and experimentally induced animal models, show clearly that genetic factors are involved in the aetiology of the autoimmune process. Thus, there is a strong family history of autoimmunity, and significant correlations can be demonstrated in individual patients and in population studies with certain HLA haplotypes encoded by the MHC genes (see Section 1.3.1 on MHC and disease). The patterns of disease inheritance do not follow simple Mendelian rules of genetics. In the case of monozygotic twins the concordance for an established autoimmune disorder such as type I diabetes mellitus is only 50 per cent. In autoimmune disease, therefore, genetic factors alone do not provide an explanation for the aetiology of the disorder. Nevertheless, current evidence strongly suggests that certain genes and their expressed products (especially those encoded in the MHC) in association with environmental factors (such as microorganisms) result in the induction of autoimmunity (see Section 1.3.1).

The HLA antigens, especially the class II molecules (DR, DQ, and DP), when aberrantly expressed on non-immune cells are thought to act as triggers and/or perpetuators of autoimmune responses. Hence, endocrine epithelial cells, if they aberrantly express class II HLA antigens, may unwittingly present their self antigens complexed with the aberrant class II HLA molecules. Such cells may behave initially as surrogate APCs and subsequently as targets for the deleterious anti-self T cell responses generated. The T cell (TCR) thus both 'sees' and is triggered by 'aberrant self'. Some authorities suggest that environmental agents such as viruses may trigger aberrant expression of HLA molecules on infected cells, or conceivably infected cells may initially excite a T lymphocyte response. The infiltrating T cells then release lymphokines, such as IFN-γ or TNF, which have been demonstrated *in vitro* to induce HLA molecules on cells which do not normally express the molecules or express them at very low levels.

Immune defects. Various abnormalities within the immune system may contribute to the induction of autoimmune responses. Patients with rare deficiences of the early components of the complement system (see Section 1.5) have an increased incidence of autoimmune disorders. Patients with a deficiency of immunoglobulin A (approximately 1 in 500 of the population) show an increased incidence of autoimmunity. It is postulated that these deficiencies are associated with a lack of the protective mechanisms normally directed to preventing autoimmunity. The majority of patients seen with autoimmune disorders do not have such obvious immune defects. Defects in functional T 'suppressor cells' have been repeatedly demonstrated in human and animal autoimmune studies, although the cloning of such cells has proved elusive.

Old age is well known to be associated with an increased incidence of autoantibody responses, accompanied by a loss of $CD4^+$ and $CD8^+$ T cells. A defect in $CD8^+$ 'suppressor cells' can be readily interpreted as permissive for the induction of B cell autoantibodies (a breaking of clonal anergy). The difficulty in this area is to define whether detectable immune defects are primary or secondary contributors to the state of autoimmunity.

Hormonal factors. It is well documented that after puberty, there is a significantly increased susceptibility to connective tissue autoimmunity in females compared with males. This could represent the effects of oestrogen and/or permissive alleles on the X chromosome. Current evidence indicates that oestrogen, and many other endocrine hormones, can directly modulate the action of lymphocytes. Thus, receptors for testosterone and for thymic hormones are shown to be expressed on $CD8^+$ T cells, and the functions of such cells are enhanced by receptor occupancy by the appropriate hormone. Contrastingly, oestrogen has been shown to down-regulate the reactivity of $CD8^+$ T cells which thus facilitates the expression of autoimmunity in females. This simplistic interpretation of hormonal effects is inadequate, because diseases such as ankylosing spondylitis (considered to be autoimmune) has a male predominance. The role of hormones in the expression of autoimmunity is far from clear.

Environmental factors. The role of *microorganisms* as triggers for autoimmunity is still a matter for debate. There is not a simple correlation of infection with autoimmunity but microorganisms, or their products, may induce autoimmunity in individuals with an appropriate immune, genetic, and hormonal background. Microorganisms may share molecular similarity (molecular mimicry) with self molecules of some individuals, and thus perturb the organisms homeostasis without an appropriate induction of protective immunity.

Research evidence also indicates that various ubiquitous organisms, such as mycobacteria, possess glycoproteins which cross-react strongly with certain cellular 'heat shock proteins'. Immune reactions to such molecules appear to correlate with certain rheumatic autoimmune disorders. It has long been known that some antigens of particular streptococcal serotypes cross-react with heart antigen, and in appropriate individuals, infection with streptococci has resulted in the induction of rheumatic fever. Other microorganisms, such as *Epstein–Barr virus*, can be shown to act as polyclonal activators of B cells, thus bypassing the need for T helper cells. By circumventing the need for T 'help', such organisms could contribute to the overcoming of clonal anergy.

Drugs, such as penicillamine, which are well documented as inducers of autoimmunity, may adsorb on to cells and alter the structure of self molecules, so that they become antigenic.

Clearly, environmental trauma, which leads to the release of sequestered antigens (e.g., in the eye, heart or urogenital tract), can lead to the induction of autoimmune responses. Interestingly, the autoimmune responses which commonly follow trauma and surgery are transient and illustrate that induction of autoantibodies may not be sufficient in itself for induction of clinical autoimmunity; other 'factors' in the individual's immunogenetic background may be required.

1.6.3 Immune suppression

The adaptive immune response is generally useful, protective, and self-regulatory. Nevertheless, in some situations the response can be seen as inappropriate and harmful, as in autoimmunity, or undesirable, as in transplantation rejection. Immune suppressive regimens are used in clinical practice to overcome excessive and prolonged immune responses. The ultimate goal of immune suppression is to inhibit selectively the specific responding lymphocyte clones (T and B), leaving intact other clones and effector mechanisms which are normally useful and protective. Such a goal is far from being realized.

Attempts at suppression have progressed from the use of non-specific drugs to the recent attempts using cell-specific monoclonal antibodies.

Outlined below are some immunosuppressive agents employed in current clinical practice together with an outline of some experimental procedures which in the next few years may play an important part in clinical medicine.

Drugs

Major immunosuppressive drugs in current clinical usage include cortico-steroids, azathioprine and other thiopurines, alkylating agents such as cyclophosphamide and chlorambucil, and the novel agent Cyclosporin A (CsA). All of these agents, to varying degrees, have the drawback of suppressing the patient's immune system widely and non-specifically. Hence, the individual's defences against bacterial, fungal, and viral infections are weakened. Prolonged usage of such agents is also associated with an increased incidence of certain types of malignancies. Current evidence suggests that this latter risk is much less with CsA when used as a single agent. Another difficulty in defining the immunosuppressive role of drugs is due to their far-reaching effects on cells and systems, other than those directly related to the specific immune response. Steroids inhibit substantially the inflammatory response. They markedly affect the prostaglandin synthetic pathways and hence modulate the effectors of inflammation. They affect the biological behaviour of polymorphonuclear leucocytes, e.g., by stabilizing their lysosomal membranes, and induce a neutrophilia (Table 1.8). Steroids have also been shown to have inhibitory effects on the production of IL-1 and IL-2. They significantly alter the trafficking of lymphocytes resulting in an apparent lymphopenia. This is due, in man, mainly to bone marrow sequestration of blood CD4$^+$ T cells, rather than to a lymphocytolysis which is seen with steroid therapy in some experimental animals. Table 1.8 summarizes some of the common immunosuppressive and anti-inflammatory effects of steroids. The prolonged usage of steroids has many well-documented undesirable side-effects, apart from increased susceptibility to infections, and includes aggravation

Table 1.8. Effect of steroids

Inflammation	↓	Prostaglandin synthesis
	↓	Neutrophil enzyme release
	↑	Immature forms of neutrophils
	↑	Stabilization of lysosomal membranes
Cell functions	↓	T cell IL-2 production
	↓	Macrophages and APC
	↓↓	Chemotaxis, IL-1 and IFN-γ production
	↓	Bactericidal activity
Cell trafficking	↓	CD4$^+$ T cells
	→	CD8$^+$ T cells (as seen in blood)
	↓	Monocytes

and induction of osteoporosis, diabetes, cataracts, and Cushingoid reactions, to name but a few.

Cyclophosphamide (Cy) and related drugs interfere with DNA replication and are particularly effective against rapidly dividing cells (hence its myelotoxicity), including proliferating lymphocyte clones. Cy has been shown to reduce antibody production and delayed type hypersensitivity (DTH) reactions. In experimental systems, the administration of Cy before, at or after antigen administration can have effects ranging from marked immune suppression to striking immune enhancement. Unlike steroids, Cy has little direct anti-inflammatory effect. It is becoming increasingly apparent that apart from its alkylating role, Cy has considerable modulating effects on cells involved in the immune response. Thus in animal systems, Cy has been shown to have relatively greater effects on suppressor lymphocytes. It can, when used with immunization protocols, potentiate natural killer cell activities (some of the NK cells being able to induce 'suppressor' reactions *in vivo*), as well as having cytotoxic effects. The mechanisms of action of Cy are currently under intensive investigation, and will probably yield information defining newer roles for this long-established drug (see Chapter 7). Clinically, apart from its well-defined role in the treatment of various solid and haematological cancers, Cy is indicated in the treatment of Wegener's disease (a presumed autoaggressive immune disorder) and in ablative regimens prior to bone marrow transplantation.

Cyclosporin A (CsA) is a naturally occurring fungal metabolite. It was purified in 1973 and the first report of its immunosuppressive properties appeared in 1976. In the subsequent decade CsA became established as the primary immunosuppressive agent used in the prevention of graft rejection (see Chapter 2). Currently, CsA is being investigated as a potential drug in the clinical management of some autoimmune disorders, especially insulin-dependent diabetes mellitus (IDDM) and rheumatoid arthritis.

The main effect of CsA, established from *in vitro* experiments, is its inhibition of IL-2 production by $CD4^+$ T cells. Thus, CsA affects $CD4^+$ T cell-dependent proliferative responses, especially primary CMI responses (and DTH), and T cell-dependent antibody responses. NK cell proliferation, which is in part dependent on IL-2, is said to be also adversely affected by CsA. Currently, *in vivo* experiments indicate that the *in vitro* findings are insufficient to explain many of the effects of CsA. In humans, the immune suppressive effects of CsA appear to require its continuous usage, in marked contrast to some animal experiments where a short course of CsA administration can result in long-term immunosuppression (tolerance). The need for long-term usage of CsA in man is not without side-effects, the main problem being nephrotoxicity. The use of CsA, its side-effects, and drug monitoring in the context of transplantation, are documented in Chapter 2.

Preliminary studies using CsA in autoimmune disorders, such as chronic autoimmune uveitis and IDDM, has also demonstrated unacceptable levels of renal toxicity, and lesser degrees of hepatotoxicity. In young children in the IDDM studies, abnormal facies associated with CsA therapy were documented. Undoubtedly, CsA represents a major advance as a drug showing some degree of selective immunosuppression (affecting mainly T cell activation), but much more work is needed to define the mechanism of its actions, if it is to have a wider usage as an immunosuppressant outside the field of transplantation.

Antigens and antibodies as immune therapeutic agents

Research has established that administration of purified antigen, depending on its dose and route of administration, and age of animal, can result in suppression of immune reactivity rather than inducing humoral or cell-mediated immune responses. The phenomenon of antigen-induced immunosuppression has always been more difficult to produce with established immune responses, compared with primary antigenic stimulation. In clinical practice, suppression of established immune responses is often required. Due to the fact that, in autoimmunity, the specific exciting antigen usually is not known, or in transplantation the antigen is complex and important epitopes are ill-defined, the use of specific antigen immunosuppression in clinical medicine accordingly is exceedingly rare. The best example of the practical use of specific antigen-induced immune suppression is found in the treatment of type I hypersensitivity ('allergic') states. In some type I conditions, the antigen(s) are fairly well defined, e.g., in some forms of pollen-induced hay fever and house dust mite-associated allergic rhinitis. Purified antigens, which may or may not be partly altered by chemical or physical treatments and injected using standard protocols, can in some patients result in suppression of the associated IgE-mediated type I hypersensitivity state (Section 1.7). National and international agreed schemes and protocols have been produced for a limited number of such antigen-specific immunosuppressive therapies.

Experimental evidence is emerging (using gene transfection and expression in 'carrier cells') suggesting that complex antigens, such as those involved in organ rejection (i.e., HLA molecules), may ultimately be used in antigen-induced immune suppression systems. Allied experiments, using purified protein antigens administered with MABs directed to important molecules, such as the CD4 epitopes, have also indicated the possibility of relatively specific immune suppression. Additionally, recent experiments using antibodies against cell adhesion molecules (I-CAM, LFA1, CD2, and LFA3) and also against 'activation antigens' (IL-2 receptors and T cell-associated HLA-DR) have been shown to significantly down-regulate immune responses. These approaches are currently in their infancy, but eventually should provide new insights into the mechanisms and permit the therapeutic application of more selective immune suppression.

Monoclonal antibodies alone have already an established, albeit very limited, role in immune suppression in clinical practice. Thus, the use of murine MABs to CD3 (notably OKT3) is an accepted form of treatment for allograft rejection, which is unresponsive to the standard drug suppressive therapies. Polyclonal, and more latterly MAB, anti-rhesus D (RhD) antibodies administered to RhD negative mothers, has been shown to provide prophylaxis against haemolytic disease of the newborn. The mechanisms of antibody-induced immunosuppression are not clear, but experimental evidence indicates a role for antigen sequestration, suppressive anti-idiotypic receptor interactions, modulation of crucial lymphocyte subsets, and augmentation of suppressive effector reactions such as ADCC.

Antibody-induced immunosuppression is also being demonstrated and exploited in the treatment of certain autoimmune-associated haematological disorders, such as some forms of idiopathic thrombocytopenic purpura, autoimmune neutropenia, and aplastic anaemia. Clearly, the mechanisms of antibody-induced immune suppression need to be elucidated if such manœuvres are to occupy an important therapeutic role in clinical practice. One problem with using mouse MABs *in vivo* is that the human immune system recognizes the mouse immunoglobulin as a foreign antigen and generates an appropriate antibody response. The resultant human anti-mouse antibody results in the formation of immune complexes, which shorten the effective *in vivo* half-life and limit the repeated therapeutic use of the mouse MABs. As the V region in the Fab portion (see Fig. 1.9) of the MABs possess the desired specificities used in antibody therapy, new manœuvres are being tried to overcome the problems of the human anti-mouse response. One approach is the use of enzyme-treated mouse MABs, whereby most of the antigenic Fc fragment is removed before *in vivo* administration. The generated Fab fragments retain the desirable V region antibody specificity. This approach, however, is only partially successful, because some of the effector reactions associated with the mouse Fc region are desirable for therapeutic efficacy. A more elegant approach is the recent use of genetic engineering techniques to splice the DNA encoding the desired mouse V region specificity on to the DNA encoding the remainder of a human immunoglobulin (Ig). This generated hetero-immunoglobulin fulfils all the desired properties of a therapeutic antibody. Thus, mice can be immunized against any antigen, the use of which would be unethical in humans. The DNA encoding the mouse antibody specificity (V regions) can be isolated, and spliced on to the DNA of a standard human Ig (the normal human V region having been removed). The human Ig Fc region, ensures the presence of effector characteristics (e.g., complement fixation, Fc receptor binding) without undesirable Fc antigenicity in human recipients.

1.6.4 Newer immune modulators

FK-506 is a macrolide antibiotic, obtained from a soil fungus, *Streptomyces tsukubaensis*, which has demonstrated remarkable immunosuppressive properties. It is structurally distinct from CsA, yet it shares some of its properties, including inhibition of lymphokine production by activated lymphocytes and a relative lack of myelotoxicity. On a molar basis, FK-506 appears significantly more potent than CsA, and experiments have suggested that it will act synergistically with CsA *in vitro* and *in vivo*. Its anti-T cell effect results in profound suppression of CMI and of T cell-dependent humoral responses. Severe side-effects have been documented in some animal species; the situation in humans is currently under investigation. At the present time, the future clinical role of FK-506 is undefined, but preliminary evidence suggests that it may have a major role to play as either a potent single immunosuppressive agent or in conjunction with other immunosuppressive drugs.

Cytokines obtained by recombinant DNA technology, including GM-CSF, M-CSF, and IL-2, have already been used to enhance the production of cells which help to improve the performance of patients whose defences are impaired. Undoubtedly, much more use will be made of such precisely defined agents (see Section 1.4 and Chapter 7).

Newer adjuvants, such as ISCOMS (see Section 1.2.4) and muramyl dipeptide, can lead to a non-specific boost of T and B lymphocyte responses, and unlike Freund's adjuvant, appear to be acceptable for use in humans (see Chapter 4).

NK and LAK cells already have a defined role as anti-cancer cell agents (see previous Section 1.5 and Chapter 3). Recent experiments have indicated that they may also have a significant anti-bacterial and anti-viral role. The use of NK and LAK cell activities, enhanced by using drugs and cytokines, such as IL-2 and IFN-γ, may have clinical relevance for surgeons and physicians combating severe sepsis associated with immune depression.

1.7 Immunopathological processes—hypersensitivity (types I–IV) and tissue damage

Humoral and cell-mediated immunity (CMI) usually are beneficial and protective host defence mechanisms. Nevertheless, situations occur where either one or both reactions can result in more tissue damage than protection. The mechanistic and descriptive cataloguing of such immunopathology is embodied in the term *hypersensitivity*, which was originally crystallized by Gell and Coombs as type I–IV hypersensitivity reactions.

Table 1.9. Antigens associated with hypersensitivity reactions

Entrinsic
Bacteria, viruses, fungi
Allergens—pollen, dust mites, foods, drugs
Mismatched tissues and cells

Intrinsic
Red cells, leucocytes, platelets

Organ specific
  Endocrine glands—thyroid, adrenal, etc.
  Skeletal muscle, gastric mucosa

Non-organ specific
  Immunoglobulin
  Antigens of nuclei
Smooth muscle and mitochondrial antigens

Types I, II, and III are mediated mainly by antibodies and type IV by agents of CMI. These reactions can be directed against extrinsic antigens or autoantigens (Table 1.9). The unifying feature is that once the specific reactants are triggered they recruit complement, polymorphs, and other leucocytes, which act as the mediators of damage. Although the description of type I–IV conveniently summarizes the mechanisms of the reactions, the classification does not consider the possible aetiological factors.

Outlined below is the classification of type I–IV hypersensitivity reactions, with appropriate clinical examples.

Type I hypersensitivity is also referred to as immediate hypersensitivity. Within this grouping can be found disorders (which in common parlance are called 'allergic' reactions) such as hay fever, asthma, and anaphylaxis associated with reactions to agents, such as halothane, penicillin, and other drugs. Type I reactions are due to IgE antibodies, which are bound in high numbers to the membrane receptors (termed Fcε) of tissue mast cells and blood basophils, see Fig. 1.17(a). Contrastingly, the amount of IgE in blood is very low compared with the other isotypes.

Although everyone produces IgE antibodies, it is evident upon examination of family histories of 'allergy' sufferers, that there is a genetic predisposition for developing type I hypersensitivity. The inheritance and exhibition of the hypersensitivity phenotype is denoted by the term 'atopy', the hypersensitive individual being termed an 'atopic'. Such individuals may or may not have raised IgE levels, they usually have a strong family history of type I allergic reactions and often have multiple IgE antibodies to several different antigens. The basis of their genetic predisposition is far from clear, but in some cases an association with certain HLA phenotypes is documented. Also, the induction of IgE antibodies is highly dependent on and is controlled by various immunoregulatory T lymphocytes. Aberrations in T cells have been clearly documented in experimental models of Type I hypersensitivity; such evidence is being activately sought in humans. Clinically, it has long been known that psychological factors, 'stressors', can precipitate or intensify 'allergic' type I reactions. Recent evidence has demonstrated that neuroendocrine-linked reactions can clearly trigger type I reactions in highly sensitized experimental animals, apparently without the presence of the allergen!

From Fig. 1.17(a) it can be seen that when the 'antigen' cross-links (bridges) two IgE molecules on the surface of the mast cell, a stimulatory transmembrane signal is sent, which ultimately 'activates' the mast cell to release its preformed stored granules and to synthesize further 'mediators'. It is the released products of the tissue mast cells and of basophils in blood, which lead to the dramatic clinical manifestations of type I reactions. The released mediators are potent stimulators of acute inflammation, and also act on smooth muscle and the blood vascular endothelium. The release of the preformed mediators account for the rapid time course of type I reactions which occur within minutes of exposure to the antigen (also called the allergen).

Current laboratory tests designed to document type I reactions include PRIST for total IgE; RAST and ELISA-based systems for specific IgE antibodies (see Chapter 9). For suspected type I reactions to anaesthetic agents, such as halothane, suxamethonium, and procainamide as well as

(a) Type I hypersensitvity

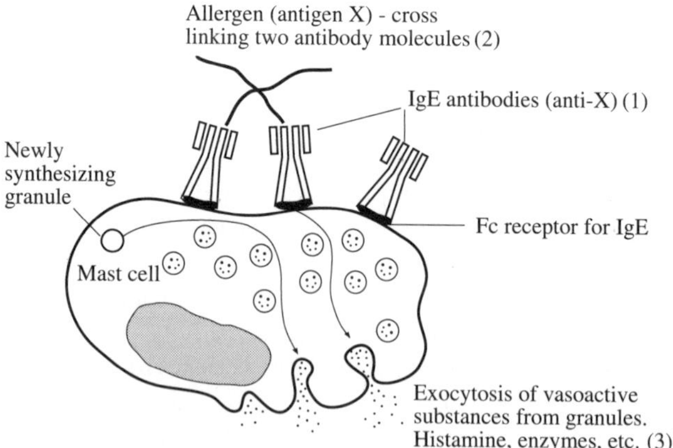

Fig. 1.17. Hypersensitivity reactions: type I–IV.

(b) Type II hypersensitivity

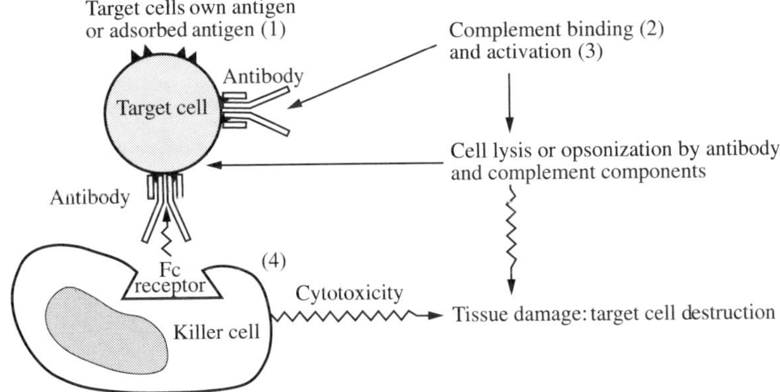

(c) Type III hypersensitivity

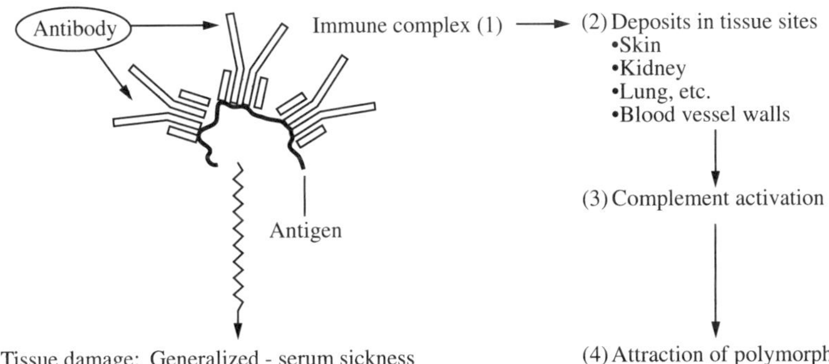

(d) Type IV hypersensitivity

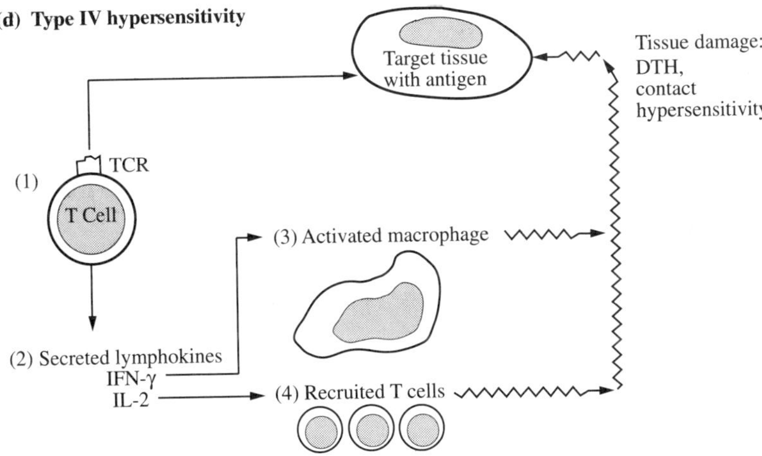

Fig. 1.17. *cont'd.*

to other drugs, the current tests are far from ideal and are of unproven value. Depending on the methods employed for data collection, e.g., population surveys, anaesthetic, surgical, and post-mortem records, the incidence of such type I reactions to drugs are variously reported (in different surveys) from approximately 1: 400 to less than 1: 10 000!

Treatment of type I reactions is based ideally on prophylaxis/prevention. Drugs which antagonize various pathways involved in type I reactions have proved extremely useful, together with agents which help to inhibit or modify the damage caused to the target organs. Sodium chromoglycate (Intal) acts, at various biochemical levels, on the mast cell to inhibit its reaction to the allergen-IgE signal of activation and its consequent release of mediators. β_1 and β_2 adrenergic agonists (isoprenaline, salbutamol) help to relax the smooth muscle and vascular spasm induced by mast cell mediators. Steroids, administered locally and systemically, have a broad-based 'anti-inflammatory reaction' against many agents and mediators involved in the type I reaction. Attempts at hyposensitization, by injecting various forms of purified allergens, to date, has proved clinically less successful (with a few striking exceptions) than predicted from basic research. Undoubtedly, part of the problem is inadequate purification and definition of the appropriate 'allergens', and lack of knowledge of the best injection protocols with respect to timing and dosage. It is to be hoped that some of these problems will be overcome in the near future.

Type II hypersensitivity involves antibodies directed to and reacting with antigens which are part of a cell membrane. The antigen may be an integral membrane component, or can be of extrinsic origin that becomes adsorbed to the cell (e.g., drugs). The result of such a siting is that antibodies, mainly of the IgG and IgM class, after reacting with the cell membrane antigen, recruit and activate effectors such as complement or cells with appropriate Fc receptors. The latter then mediate cellular and tissue damage at the site of the bound antibodies, see Fig. 1.17(b). In some situations, if the antibodies bind to a functional receptor (antigen) on the cell membrane, it may trigger the associated cell function. An important example of this stimulatory damaging type II reaction is that involved in the pathogenesis of Graves disease. The IgG autoantibody, termed long-acting thyroid stimulator (LATS) or more appropriately thyroid-stimulating immunoglobulin (TSI), binds to the TSH receptor on the surface of thyroid cells. The resulting enhanced activity of the thyroid cells leads to excessive and continued release of the thyroid hormones and clinical hyperthyroidism. Some authorities have tried to classify 'stimulatory' type II reactions, into a separate (but perhaps unnecessary) type V category.

Some well-known examples of Type II reactions include reactions against blood cells in mismatched transfusions, autoimmune haemolytic anaemias, drug-induced reactions to blood cells, and haemolytic disease of the newborn. Certain autoimmune diseases have type II reactions as the main immunopathological basis of damage, e.g., myasthenia gravis and Goodpasture's syndrome.

Type III hypersensitivity involves preformed antibody interacting with antigen, the resultant *immune complexes* mediating tissue damage when they precipitate in tissue sites. The deposited complexes recruit and activate complement and effector cells which can result in severe tissue damage. Classical examples of type III systemic reactions are embodied by the 'serum sickness' syndromes, and the more localized form of Type III by the so-called 'Arthus reaction', see Fig. 1.17(c). The reactions triggered by the immune complexes are usually manifested as clinical inflammation, 6 to 24 hours following exposure to the antigen. Serum sickness historically was associated with treatments, such as the administration of passive antisera (e.g., horse immunoglobulin to treat patients exposed to the tetanus bacilli). The patient, over a period of time (4–10 days), develops high levels of anti-horse immunoglobulin antibodies. These form immune complexes in the systemic circulation with the declining levels of the administered horse proteins, the resultant immune complex-mediated inflammation being manifested as an acute serum sickness syndrome. The patients develop urticaria, arthralgia, and glomerulonephritis, due to the soluble immune complexes precipitating in associated tissue sites. In the Arthus reaction, the preformed antibodies interact with antigens, which are present in high concentration in local sites, e.g., the dermis, the bronchial tree. The resultant local concentrations of immmune complexes induce severe localized immune inflamation. Well-known examples of type III reactions include some forms of immune complex-induced glomerulonephritis and dermatitis, associated with extrinsic antigens (microorganisms) and with autoantigens in autoimmune diseases, such as SLE.

Type IV reactions, which are associated with specific T lymphocytes, see Fig. 1.7(d), are interpreted as excessive tissue-damaging CMI reactions, the clinical description of which is termed delayed type hypersensitivity (DTH), due to the time taken for maximal clinical expression, i.e., 2–3 days compared with the minutes to hours for type I, II, and III reactions. As described in Section 1.3.3, sensitized T lymphocytes recognize antigen appropriately and secrete lymphokines which attract other T lymphocytes and macrophages to the antigen site. The crucial factors which result in this CMI becoming overtly pathological rather than physiologically protective, are not fully elucidated. Undoubtedly, in some situations it is due to the nature of the antigen, which persists because it is biologically non-degradeable (e.g., metal ions, resistant intracellular organisms) and thus leads to continued and excessive stimulation of CMI. Some well-known DTH type IV reactions include certain viral-induced skin rashes, the iatrogenic Mantoux test, dermatitis associated with 'allergy' to metals and industrial chemicals, and the tuberculoid form of leprosy.

Although the hypersensitivity tissue-damaging reactions can be conveniently described in the type I–IV compartments, *in vivo* such separations are less readily discernable and are a gross over-simplification. Thus, the patient manifesting a severe and protracted asthmatic attack triggered by a type I reaction may, with time, develop concurrently elements of type II and III reactions. Similarly, many highly sensitized patients experiencing type IV reactions can, on examination, be shown to have elements of type II hypersensitivity reactions. The clarification of the *in vivo* interactions of the various elements of hypersensitivity reactions will lead to more efficient forms of therapy, particularly combinational treatment, and ultimately prophylaxis.

References and further reading

Chapel, H. and Haeney, M. (1988). *Essentials of clinical Immunology* (2nd edn). Blackwell, Oxford.

Roitt, I.M., Brostoff, J., and Male, D. (1989). *Immunology* (2nd edn). Churchill Livingstone, London.

Stites, D.P. and Terr, I.A. (ed.) (1987). *Basic and clinical immunology* (7th edn). Appleton and Lange, Norwalk, Conneticut.

2
Transplantation immunology

R.F.M. Wood

2.1 The human MHC

The key to transplantation immunology is to achieve an understanding of the major histocompatibility complex (MHC). Genes within all nucleated human cells control the expression of molecules which project outwards from the cell surface. These cell surface antigens have developed through evolution as important self markers to ensure that the immune system is confined to attacking foreign targets. The human MHC is located on the short arm of chromosome 6. The main loci are shown in Fig. 2.1. The A

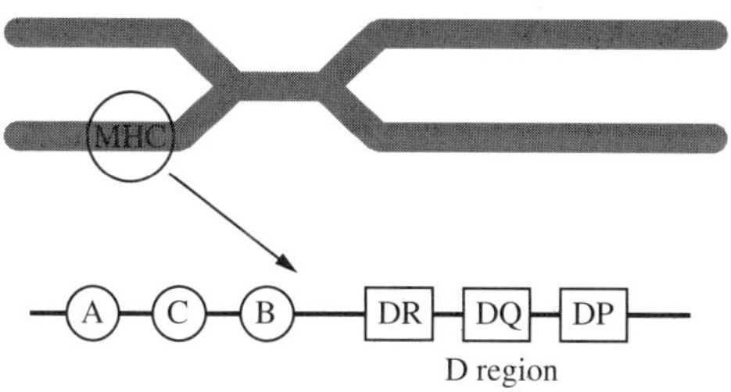

Fig. 2.1. The human MHC loci on chromosome 6. MHC, major histocompatibility complex.

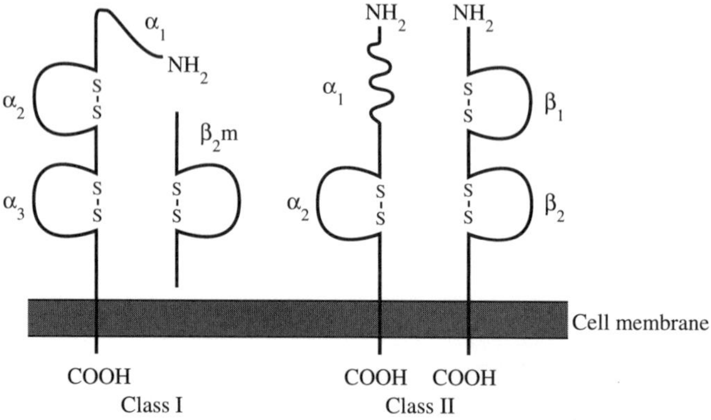

Fig. 2.2. The structure of class I and II antigens.

and B loci control the expression of so-called class I products on the cell surface while the loci in the D region control class II antigen expression. The characteristic structure of class I and class II antigens is shown in Fig. 2.2 (see also Chapter 1, Section 1.3.1).

2.2 HLA antigens

The cell surface products are known as human leucocyte antigens (HLAs). This is because they were first identified on white blood cells. However, as indicated above, these antigens are expressed on all nucleated cells. The level of expression varies and this applies particularly to class II products which have a much more limited expression than class I antigens. For example, in the peripheral blood, class II antigens are normally expressed on B lymphocytes but minimally on T lymphocytes. Each individual has a 'phenotype' which is made up of two 'haplotypes'—the genetic information on each short arm of chromosome 6. Individuals inherit one complete haplotype from each parent. This genetic information is usually defined in terms of the serologically determined A, B, and DR loci. There are 23 A locus alleles, 49 B locus alleles, and 16 DR locus alleles (Table 2.1). Although there is, therefore, almost an infinite number of different 'tissue types' certain combinations of antigens occur with relatively high frequency.

2.3 Tissue typing

A close affinity between donor and recipient will reduce the stimulus to the host immune system and lessen the rejection reaction. Tissue typing for HLA antigens, therefore, has been developed as a means of selecting the best matched recipient for any given donor. This applies particularly

Table 2.1. The A, B, and DR specificities used in clinical tissue typing

A	B		DR
A1	B5	Bw50	DR1
A2	B7	B51	DR2
A3	B8	Bw52	DR3
A9	B12	Bw53	DR4
A10	B13	Bw54	DR5
A11	B14	Bw55	DRw6
Aw19	B15	Bw56	DR7
A23	B16	Bw57	DRw8
A24	B17	Bw58	DR9
A25	B18	Bw59	DRw10
A26	B21	Bw60	DRw11
A28	Bw22	Bw61	DRw12
A29	B27	Bw62	DRw13
A30	B35	Bw63	DRw14
A31	B37	Bw64	DRw15
A32	B38	Bw65	DRw16
Aw33	B39	Bw67	DRw17
Aw34	B40	Bw70	DRw18
Aw36	Bw41	Bw72	
Aw43	Bw42	Bw73	DRw52
Aw66	B44	Bw75	
Aw68	B45	Bw76	DRw53
Aw69	Bw46	Bw77	
Aw74	Bw47		
	Bw48	Bw4	
	B49	Bw6	

in renal transplantation (Gilks *et al.* 1987). In other forms of organ grafting, HLA matching has, so far, been precluded because of the time taken to achieve an accurate tissue type result.

Tissue typing is performed by reacting lymphocytes from the individual under test with a range of HLA anti-sera. The anti-sera are obtained from pregnant women who have produced antibodies to specific HLA determinants on fetal cells which are of paternal origin. In tissue typing cadaver transplant donors it is usually difficult to prepare a good B lymphocyte suspension from the peripheral blood. Therefore, a specimen of spleen is removed at the time of organ harvest and used as a source of lymphocytes. A crude cell suspension in tissue culture medium is prepared from the splenic tissue and layered on to a density gradient solution in centrifuge tubes. Spinning forces debris and red blood cells to the bottom of the tube leaving a layer of lymphocytes at the interface between the tissue culture medium and the density gradient solution (see Chapter 9, p. 185.) The lymphocytes are washed, resuspended, and plated out in tissue typing trays. These pre-prepared trays, known as micro-titre plates, have wells with each one containing a different anti-serum to a known HLA specificity. Using a micro-pipette, 100 μl of cell suspension (approximately 20 000 cells) and 100 μl of rabbit complement are added to each well of the plate. The dye is only taken up by dead cells which have been killed by the combined action of anti-serum and complement. By studying the patterns of cytotoxicity the tissue type of the individual can be determined (see Chapter 9, Section 9.4 on tissue typing methods).

National and regional transplant organizations keep computerized records of the tissue types of all their potential transplant recipients. Hence, a rank order of the most appropriate recipients, for a particular donor organ, can readily be determined.

2.4 Immune responses to foreign HLA antigens

2.4.1 Antibody responses

The recognition of foreign class I and class II products stimulates both humoral and cellular immune responses. As mentioned above, the humoral response to foreign fetal antigens generates circulating anti-HLA antibodies in the mother's blood. Antibodies can also be formed against HLA antigens expressed on platelets and white cells in transfused blood. In organ transplant recipients, antibodies develop against mis-matched HLA determinants expressed on donor endothelial cells or 'passenger' leucocytes within the donor organ. These antibodies tend to fix to target tissue within the graft and, therefore, can be difficult to detect. However, if the organ is removed because of rejection there is usually a rapid rise in the titre of antibody in the peripheral blood.

2.4.2 Cell-mediated rejection

Although antibody responses are of undoubted importance in transplantation it is the classic cell-mediated response which is the dominant feature of the immune reaction to an organ allograft. The hypothesis of a cell-mediated reaction to transplanted tissue was first propounded by Gibson and Medawar in 1943. They carried out detailed histological studies on skin grafts used to treat a young woman with severe burns. The grafted skin had been obtained from the girl's brother. The initial set of 'pinch' skin grafts placed on the burned area gradually deteriorated and a second set of grafts was employed. These subsequent grafts were shed much more rapidly than the initial set. After careful histological studies, Gibson and Medawar proposed that this 'second set' reaction was due to actively acquired immunity on the part of the recipient. These clinical observations formed the basis of a series of elegant animal experiments in the mid-1940s in which Medawar established the predominantly cellular nature of allograft rejection. It became clear that the lymphocyte was the cell primarily responsible for orchestrating the rejection response. In the early 1950s, it was demonstrated that transplantation immunity could be transferred from one animal to another by an injection of sensitized lymphocytes. Lymphocytes were harvested from a mouse of strain A, which had rejected a skin graft from an animal of a different inbred strain (B). These sensitized A-strain lymphocytes were administered to another A-strain mouse, which had just received a B-strain skin graft. The graft was rejected in an accelerated fashion.

It is now clear that the sensitization process is triggered by the recognition of foreign antigens by host lymphocytes. Following revascularization of an organ allograft small particles of antigenic material or 'passenger' donor leucocytes are washed out into the recipient circulation. This is followed by antigen presentation to T lymphocytes accompanied by the secretion of a soluble mediator – interleukin-1(IL-1). This two signal process – antigen plus IL-1 – sends a signal to the synthetic processes within the T lymphocyte causing proliferation and cell division (see Chapter 1, Section 1.3). The resultant blast cells are sometimes known as 'immunoblasts' as they have the potential to migrate to the graft and initiate the destructive process of rejection. Sensitization probably also occurs within the graft by direct contact between recipient lymphocytes and class II expressing, graft dendritic cells. Dendritic cells are so called because of their finger-like processes.

The sensitized lymphocytes produce a range of mediators known as lymphokines. They are essentially protein hormones – single chain polypeptides with no structural homology. Interleukin-2 stimulates the clonal expansion of the sensitized T cell population. Other lymphokines have the capacity to cause direct cytotoxicity to target cell in the graft without the additional help of the complement pathway. Lymphokines are also important in augmenting the inflammatory response to the graft by mobilizing other members of the white cell series. This is achieved by the secretion of chemotactic factors, and factors such as leucocyte migration inhibition factor, which have been identified in *in vitro* systems. So far, seven interleukins have been identified and the genes for them have been cloned. Interleukins 1, 2, 4, and 7 all have a major role in lymphopoiesis, whereas interleukins 3, 5, and 6 play a major role in stimulating the growth and maturation of non-lymphoid cells (see Chapter 1, Section 1.4).

T cells recognize their specific targets by means of a cell surface receptor. In addition to the class I antigens there are a number of other molecules projecting from the T cell membrane. For example, CD3 is a molecule present on the surface of virtually all mature peripheral T cells. The T cell receptor is a cell surface heterodimer closely associated with the chains of the CD3 complex. Antigen binding to the receptor site causes transduction of a signal to the synthetic machinery of the cell. In an already sensitized cell this will produce a brisk response in terms of lymphokine secretion. Prompt effector cell function can only occur when there is adequate cell-to-cell contact. The attachment between leucocytes and endothelium involves another family of heterodimeric cell surface receptor molecules—the 'integrins' or 'leucocyte adhesion molecules'. Integrin binding to the sub-endothelial matrix initiates locomotion of the cells by means of cytoskeletal proteins. The molecules also appear to function as transcellular carriers of cytokines. Outside the context of transplantation they have an important role in limiting local tissue damage and initiating repair. However, in rejection they act to amplify the inflammatory response by involving polymorphs and macrophages to add to the tissue destruction initiated by the lymphocytes.

2.4.3 Natural defence mechanisms

The elimination of extraneous antigens does not always require specific sensitization. The so-called 'natural killer' (NK) cells are capable of destroying foreign targets without prior sensitization. Their primary role is thought to be immune surveillance and the removal of aberrant cells capable of causing cancer (see Chapter 3, Section 3.4.3.) Whether they have any significant role in rejection is unclear. The numbers of NK cells remain depressed after transplantation; this may be an important factor in the increased incidence of malignancy seen in the long-term survivors of organ allografts.

2.4.4 Graft versus host disease

While the lymphocytes of the recipient are organizing themselves to attack the graft, the same process can occur in reverse, if the transplant contains a substantial amount of lymphoid tissue. This is particularly likely to occur if the recipient is already immunocompromised, is relatively immunoincompetent due to disease or is iatrogenically immunosuppressed. Graft versus host disease (GVHD) is a major concern in bone marrow transplantation. Proliferating graft lymphocytes attack liver, gut, and skin causing jaundice, diarrhoea, and skin rashes. T cell depletion of donor marrow, prior to infusion, is used to combat the problem. In organ transplantation, GVHD is not encountered in renal or heart transplantation, where there are virtually no lymphoid elements in the graft. Experimental evidence suggests that GVHD can occur in liver transplantation, but it has not proved to be a significant entity in clinical transplantation. The small bowel contains large concentrations of lymphoid tissue in the Peyer's patches and mesenteric lymph nodes, in addition to the lymphocytes in the intra-epithelial compartment. GVHD, therefore, is a major factor in intestinal transplantation. The phenomenon is well described in experimental studies and has also been recognized in some clinical cases.

2.5 Tolerance and enhancement

Ideally, rejection would be countered by manipulation of the immune system, masking the antigens of the transplant, or using suppressor mechanisms to switch off the effector response. To some extent, this has proved possible in animal models but it has yet to be achieved on a reliable and reproducible basis in man. If mammals are exposed to foreign antigens *in utero* a lifetime tolerance can be induced. This happens as a naturally occuring phenomenon in cattle. In a twin pregnancy there is cross-circulation between the placentas of the developing calves. Medawar and his colleages investigated the immunological effects of this chimerism. Skin grafts can be exchanged between twin calves with no evidence of rejection, although the individual animals have originated from separate embryos and, therefore, are genetically distinct. Transplant tolerance of this kind can be accomplished in laboratory animals by means of donor antigen pre-treatment. However, the achievement of tolerance is critically dependent upon the strain combination of the animals used, and the dosage, route, and timing of antigen administration.

'Enhancement' is the term given to immune-mediated processes which modify the rejection response. It has been demonstrated, in adoptive transfer experiments, that enhancement can be mediated by both serum factors and lymphocytes. For example, the spleen cells of rats immunosuppressed with Cyclosporin and bearing long-surviving heart grafts are capable of delaying the onset of rejection in a non-immunosuppressed animal, if administered at the time of heart grafting. In this situation, the enhancement is thought to be due to the action of 'suppressor' T cells. In human transplantation, the incidence of acute rejection diminishes after the first two to three months following grafting. This may well be due to the development of suppressor cells which subvert the potentially destructive activities of the effector cell population.

Blood transfusion emerged in the early 1970s as a potent means of achieving enhancement in clinical renal transplantation. A number of investigations were able to demonstrate a dose-response effect with higher graft survival rates in poly-transfused patients compared with those who had received only one or two units of blood. The worst results were seen in non-transfused individuals. However, with Cyclosporin-induced immunosuppression the 'blood transfusion effect' is marginal. In view of the risk of generating cytotoxic antibodies, protocols for deliberate blood transfusions in potential kidney recipients have largely been abandoned.

2.6 Immunosuppression

It has so far proved impossible to achieve reliable and specific blocking of the immune recognition and sensitization processes. Therefore, in practical terms, organ transplantation has had to rely on drug treatment aimed at suppressing the function of effector cells. Experimental work published in 1959 demonstrated the immunosuppressive potential of the anti-cancer drug, 6-mercaptopurine (6-MP). In canine renal transplant experiments, Calne *et al.* (1962) were subsequently able to demonstrate that a derivative of 6-MP, azathioprine, was a potent and effective agent in producing long-term graft survival. The suppressive effect of corticosteroid drugs had previously been described in animal models, and for the next 20 years the combination of azathioprine and steroids became the standard regimen in clinical transplantation. Although this therapy allowed renal and liver transplant programmes to become established there were major problems associated with their use. In renal transplantation, acute rejection was responsible for a 20 to 25 per cent graft failure rate within the first six months. The profound marrow depression produced by the drugs led to significant opportunistic infections, which were frequently fatal in high-risk cases. High-dose steroids caused their own problems—fragile skin, avascular necrosis of bone, hypertension, diabetes, cataract, and gastrointestinal haemorrhage. Despite extensive experimental work, the search for more specific and effective immunosuppressive drugs proved elusive. The only additional preparation of proven value was anti-lymphocyte globulin (ALG). ALG is produced by repeated injections of human lymphocytes into animals, such as horse, rabbit, or goat. The animal produces circulating polyclonal antibodies directed against cell surface markers on the human white cell. By separating the globulin fraction from the serum of the animal, and absorbing activity against red cells and platelets, an agent can be produced which is capable of causing lymphopenia when injected *in vivo*. ALG has proved a useful agent in both the initial immunosuppression of renal transplant recipients and in the treatment of acute rejection episodes. However, there can be allergic reactions to the animals protein of the preparation and this is a particular problem with ALG produced in horses. Patients who receive ALG rapidly become leucopaenic and are at risk of developing opportunistic infections. To reduce the risks to which they are exposed in the hospital environment, reverse barrier nursing should be instituted and care taken to provide food which is free from possible bacterial contamination.

2.6.1 Cyclosporin

In 1983, a more specific and effective immunosuppressive agent became commercially available—Cyclosporin—a metabolite of the fungal species

Tolypocladium inflatum Gams. Initial research demonstrated that, in laboratory mice, Cyclosporin caused significant suppression of the immune response to injections of foreign antigens. Subsequently, the potency of the drug was confirmed with the achievement of prolonged survival of renal, liver, and cardiac allografts in experimental animals. *In vitro* cellular studies have shown that Cyclosporin has a selective action on T lymphocytes. The drug does not seem to affect the binding of antigen or interleukin to the lymphocyte cell surface. It appears that Cyclosporin, probably working at an intracellular level, blocks the transmission of signals that would otherwise lead to cellular proliferation and the secretion of effector molecules. By acting at this relatively early stage in the rejection pathway, lymphocytes are prevented from orchestrating a response involving the other members of the white cell series. However, as Cyclosporin has less of a direct effect on B lymphocytes, polymorphs, and macrophages, patients are less susceptible to bacterial infection.

Despite the undoubted immunosuppressive potency of the drug the early clinical trials were beset with problems. In kidney transplant recipients, renal function failed to reach normal levels. It was assumed that this was due to inadequate control of rejection and drug dosage was increased. Paradoxically, renal function became worse. It was eventually established that Cyclosporin has potent nephrotoxic effects on the human kidney, and that improved renal function could be achieved using reduced dosage protocols. Nephrotoxicity appears to be due to an effect on the microvasculature of the kidney causing spasm of the afferent arteriole. It now seems likely that this is mediated through the prostaglandin system. There are a number of drug interactions involving Cyclosporin which are of clinical importance. Drugs which have a nephrotoxic potential of their own, for example antibiotics like gentamicin, can augment the nephrotoxicity caused by Cyclosporin. Agents such as rifampicin, isoniazid, and phenytoin potentiate the cyclo-oxygenase enzyme system within the liver, accelerating the metabolism of Cyclosporin and causing low blood levels on normal dosage regimens. Other drugs like erythromycin and ketoconazole, which suppress liver enzymes, may lead to a rapid increase in blood levels and a need to reduce Cyclosporin dosage to avoid nephrotoxicity.

2.6.2 Monoclonal antibodies

ALG is a polyclonal reagent and, therefore, active against the whole range of lymphocytes, with consequent depletion of both T and B lymphocyte subsets. The prospect of targeting therapy against specific lymphocyte subpopulations has always been attractive. In response to cellular stimulation a specific antibody is produced to each individual epitope expressed on the surface of the immunizing cells. However, despite a great deal of research effort, it proved impossible to clone the individual antibody secreting B cells and maintain them in culture. The breakthrough came with the work of Kohler and Milstein (1976). They were able to fuse antibody-producing B lymphocytes from the mouse with cells of a mouse myeloma in tissue culture. The myeloma cells had an enzyme defect and could not survive if the culture medium was deficient in certain substrates. As a result of fusion, the hybrid cells acquired a salvage enzyme pathway from the normal B lymphocytes. The hybrid cells continued to grow in substrate deficient medium while the large number of unfused myeloma cells died off. By cloning individual hybrid cells Kohler and Milstein were able to produce large quantities of pure monocloncal antibody (MAB). A wide range of antibody reagents are now available directed at determinants on human white cells. There were high hopes that MAB to lymphocyte markers might be effective immunosuppressive agents; for example, antibodies directed against the markers CD4 (helper/inducer) and CD8 (suppressor/cytotoxic) (see Chapter 1 page 33). Unfortunately, MABs, have proved rather disappointing in clinical practice. There are a number of problems associated with their use. As the MABs consist of mouse protein they, therefore, incite an antibody reaction of their own when administered to a patient. Binding of the antibody to the target cell surface does not necessarily bring about the destruction of the cell. Immunomodulation may occur with the disappearance of the cell surface marker while the cell itself continues to survive. Recently, MAB to the CD3 marker—OKT3—has been shown to be effective in reversing acute rejection crises in patients on conventional immunosuppression with azathioprine and prednisolone. The binding site for OKT3 is close to the T cell receptor. The agent undoubtedly causes lympholysis and this is manifest by febrile reactions in response to treatment. OKT3 continues to be used widely, either as part of the initial immunosuppressive protocol or as treatment for rejection.

2.7 Immunological aspects of clinical transplantation

There are three types of rejection in the clinical situation: hyperacute, acute, and chronic.

2.7.1 Hyperacute rejection

This rejection is due to the presence of preformed cytotoxic antibodies, directed at mis-matched HLA determinants expressed on graft endothelium. As indicated above, these antibodies form as a result of previous blood transfusion, pregnancy, or especially after a previous failed transplant. Antibodies are detected by screening serum samples from prospective recipients against a panel of cells from normal individuals. In highly reactive individuals it may be possible to identify the HLA determinants to which the antibodies are directed. These specificities can then be avoided when selecting an appropriate donor. A cytotoxic cross-match between donor cells and recipient serum is mandatory before proceeding with a transplant. Operation, in the presence of a positive cross-match, applies to renal transplantation. Following the release of the vascular clamps the kidney may initially become perfused, but then rapidly becomes blue and flabby, as the micro-circulation becomes occluded. Antibody binding to the endothelium activates the complement pathway causing cellular destruction. Parallel stimulation of the coagulation cascade results in platelet adhesion to the denuded surface of the glomerular capillary loops with irreversible failure of perfusion. Not all antibodies giving a positive reaction in a cross-match test will necessarily cause hyperacute rejection. Transplantation may still be possible if the reaction is due to autoantibodies, antibodies to B cells, and even some IgM anti-T cell antibodies. Characterization of the antibody causing the positive response is important and Ting (1989) has provided an algorithm for reaching the correct decision in the individual case.

2.7.2 Acute rejection

This type of rejection is the clinical manifestation of the classical cell-mediated process originally described by Medawar. The immunological changes described above are accompanied by signs of organ failure. Reduced urine output in kidney transplants, jaundice in the liver recipient, and breathlessness and signs of left ventricular failure in heart transplant patients. As acute rejection is an intense inflammatory reaction, in many instances, there is a systemic reaction with pyrexia and general malaise. Increased immunosuppressive therapy is required to bring the situation under control. Standard treatment is with three doses of 0.5 g of intravenous methyl prednisolone administered on successive days. This regimen can be repeated again after five days if there is no clinical evidence of a response. In 'steroid resistant' rejection ALG or OKT3 may be required to reverse the immune attack on the graft.

2.7.3 Chronic rejection

This rejection is characterized by a slowly progressive reduction in graft function. In patients with renal transplants there will be a gradual fall in creatinine clearance and a rise in serum creatinine. In cardiac transplant recipients, the ECG will show a reduction in voltage and in hepatic transplant patients, liver function tests will reveal evidence of progressive hepato-cellular damage. The damage to the graft is usually the result of the combination of two factors; previous acute rejection and the effects of antibodies. Chronic antibody-mediated damage causes arteriolar narrowing with re-duplication of the internal elastic lamina. The graft is slowly deprived of blood and extensive interstitial fibrosis develops.

2.8 Future developments

Molecular biological techniques have enabled the precise structure of HLA antigens to be determined, and there is a much more detailed understanding of the intracellular events leading to sensitization. It is, therefore, conceivable to consider more specific means of controlling the immune response. For example, lymphocyte targeted agents to block lymphokine production and drugs capable of inactivating cell surface molecules. In the long term it may be feasible to induce structural changes in recognition molecules which will effectively abrogate the response to foreign HLA antigens.

References and further reading

Calne, R. Y., Alexandre, G. P. J., and Murray, J. E. (1962). A study of the effects of drugs in prolonging survival of homologous renal transplants in dogs. *Annals of the New York Academy of Science*, **99**, 743–61.

Gibson, T. and Medawar, P. B. (1943). The fate of skin homografts in man. *Journal of Anatomy*, **77**, 299–310.

Gilks, W. R., Bradley, B. A., Gore, S. M., and Klouda, P. T. (1987). Substantial benefits of tissue matching in renal transplantation. *Transplantation*, **43**, 669–74.

Kohler, G. and Milstein, C. (1976). Derivation of specific antibody producing tissue culture and tumour lines by cell fusion. *European Journal of Immunology*, **6**, 511–19.

Ting, A. (1989). Positive crossmatches—when is it safe to transplant? *Transplant International*, **2**, 2–77.

3
Cancer and the immune response

O. Eremin

3.1 Introduction

Cancer, or neoplasia, is a process(es) by which the normal controlling mechanisms that regulate cell growth and differentiation are impaired, resulting in progressive, uncontrolled growth with subsequent invasion of adjacent tissues and eventual distal dissemination of malignant cells. Approximately one in five people in Western societies will die from cancer.

Although some cancers are known to arise as the result of the action of defined carcinogens (chemicals, ionizing radiations, oncogenic viruses) the aetiology of the majority of the cancers occurring in man is unknown. Recent knowledge regarding proto-oncogenes and their secreted products, and the role of various growth factors on auto- and paracrine control mechanisms has added further to our understanding of basic biological mechanisms initiating/controlling cell growth and differentiation. The explosion of knowledge in immunology has led to a better understanding of the complex interplay of the various components of host defence mechanisms and their possible anti-tumour role, both in states of established malignant disease and as a surveillance mechanism.

3.2 Immune surveillance

Eighty years ago, Ehrlich proposed the theory of immune surveillance, subsequently reformulated and expounded by Burnet in the 1960s, to explain the removal (recognition and destruction) of aberrant or neoplastic clones of cells arising as a result of spontaneous mutation or the action of carcinogens. Most tumours in man appear to arise in the absence of an overt viral or chemical carcinogen. Some of these tumours probably arise as the result of spontaneous mutations. In man, approximately 3×10^{11} cells are produced each day. It has been postulated that 1 in 10^{10} cells undergo spontaneous mutations per day. The theory has generated much debate in recent years and its relevance to the clinical problem of cancer in man is still a matter of continuing controversy. In evolutionary terms, host defence mechanisms have probably developed to deal primarily with infectious agents and anti-tumour mechanisms are a possible by-product of this beneficial survival mechanism in man.

Although it has been suggested recently that 'spontaneous tumours' may not be as frequent as previously believed, post-mortem evidence in man suggests that *in situ* malignant clones are not infrequent, particularly in certain organs, e.g. thyroid, breast. These latter findings suggest that the *in situ* change may remain occult for prolonged periods of time, and that some clones obviously regress and disappear. The factors responsible for the acquisition of more aggressive characteristics by these clones are poorly defined (see Section 3.6 and Table 3.3).

At the *in situ* stage, there may be a prominent mononuclear cell infiltrate adjacent to the tumour cells. The chemotactic factors responsible for this expansion of local macrophages, and at times lymphocytes, is unknown. The presence of such cells, particularly macrophages, may not be readily evident on routine histology but can be detected by immunohistochemical staining with specific monoclonal antibodies. The precise role of this *in situ* host response is unclear. It may function as an immune surveillance mechanism inducing tumour cell stasis (by releasing growth inhibitory factors) and thereby dormancy or be actively cytotoxic (by releasing free radicals and cytolytic enzymes) with resultant tumour cell death and regression of the malignant clones. Failure to abort progression of clonal expansion of the malignant cells could be due to a number of factors; in particular, to low levels of tumour antigen expression on the cell surface and/or 'weak' antigenicity or to 'masking' of tumour antigen by excessive membrane sialomucins, thereby resulting in an ineffective host anti-tumour response (see Fig. 3.1). This 'sneaking through' at an early stage of tumour growth is believed to hamper or prevent the host defences subsequently mounting an effective anti-tumour response against the rapidly increasing load of malignant cells and the possible induction of tolerance.

Studies in animal models suggest that immune surveillance appears to operate most effectively in animals bearing strongly immunogenic tumours, e.g., tumours induced by oncogenic viruses (Moloney sarcoma virus, polyoma virus), initiate a strong host response with the generation of tumour-specific cytotoxic lymphocytes (CTLs). The latter cells are usually

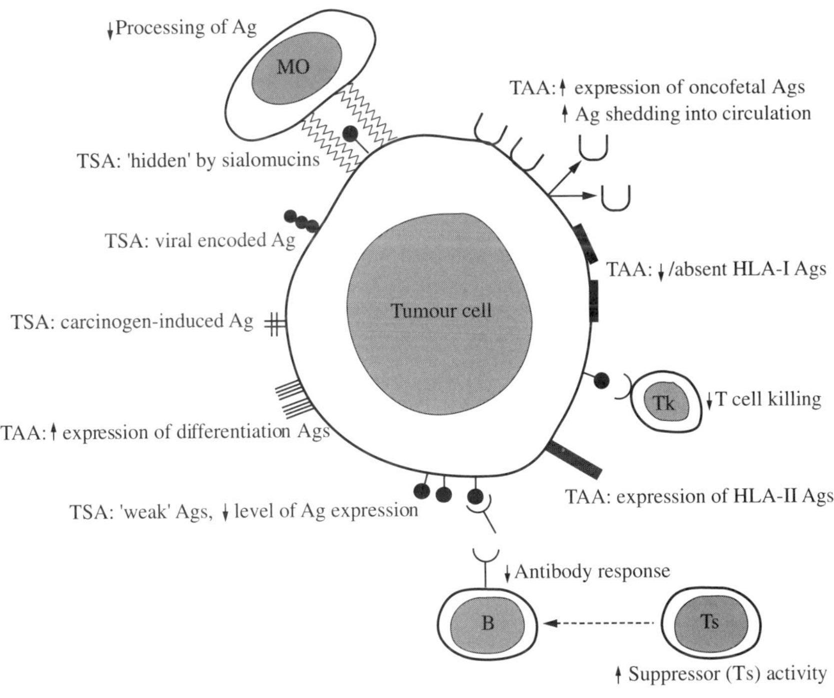

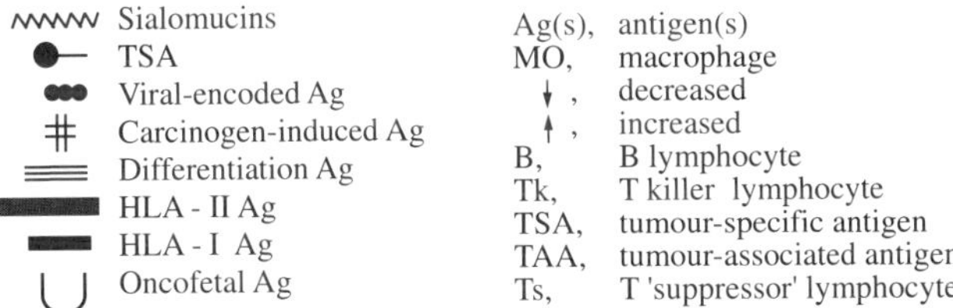

Fig. 3.1. Expression of tumour-associated antigens (TAA) and tumour-specific antigens (TSA) on the surface of a malignant cell: relationship to humoral and CMI host responses.

detected just prior to and at the time of tumour regression; the CTLs are directed against viral-induced tumour-associated antigens (TAA) and tumour-specific antigens (TSA) on the surface of the malignant cells.

Spontaneous regression, defined as the complete or partial disappearance of malignant disease following no treatment or non-curative therapy, is a rare but well-documented occurrence in man. Regression is found particularly in certain types of tumours (e.g., renal cell cancer, malignant melanoma), where there is often a prominent mononuclear (lymphocytes, macrophages) cell infiltrate within the tumours. These are the cancers that currently are showing the most efficacious responses to infusions of recombinant interleukin-2 (RIL-2) and lymphokine-activated killer (LAK) cells. It is postulated that the spontaneous regression is triggered by an *in vivo* release of cytokines (see Chapters 1 and 7).

Prolonged immunosuppression, either by pharmacological means (transplant recipients), as the result of specific viral infections (AIDS patients), or congenital defect(s) of the immune system, predispose patients to a significantly enhanced risk of developing malignant disease. The tumours which are believed to be induced by, or associated with, DNA oncoviruses or by the action of ultraviolet (UV) irradiation, include B cell lymphomas, Kaposi's sarcoma, cervical, and skin cancers. The predominant abnormality in all these patients is a severe defect of cell-mediated immunity (CMI), which is presumed to allow unopposed proliferation of DNA viruses (Epstein–Barr virus, cytomegalo-virus, human papilloma virus). Irradiation has been shown to alter immune reactivity in skin (alteration of HLA-I antigens, Langerhans cell dysfunction), and in mice (UV radiation carcinogenesis) induces the appearance of 'suppressor' cells which inhibit the development of CMI against highly immunogenic skin tumours. The evidence for the presence of immune surveillance is summarized in Table 3.1.

3.3 Tumour antigens

Early attempts to investigate anti-tumour responses in animals were frustrated by ignorance of the existence and role of histocompatibility antigens

Table 3.1. Evidence in support of immune surveillance

Biological	The relative frequency (1:10^{10}) of spontaneous mutations – malignant/aberrant clones
Pathological	The not infrequent incidence of occult *in situ* carcinoma in certain organs
Clinical	1. Severe and prolonged immunosuppression (congenital and acquired) is associated with an increase in certain types of tumour 2. 'Spontaneous' regression of malignant disease – rare but well documented
Experimental	1. T cell regression of virally induced tumours (animals) by specific T killer cells 2. NK cell – incidence of spontaneous tumours not increased in thymectomized or congenitally athymic mice

and their importance in recognition and effector responses, and by the lack of inbred strains (syngeneic) of mice. In the 1940s, it was shown that inbred mice could be immunized against a tumour that developed in a mouse of the same inbred strain. A decade later, it was demonstrated, with a methyl cholanthrene-induced tumour, that the growth of such a tumour as a transplant in a mouse, followed by its subsequent surgical removal, rendered the animal resistant to further innoculations of cells from the same tumour. Working with a similar model, others showed that the mouse was able to accept skin from a syngeneic donor (without mounting a rejection of the graft) but not tumour cells. These experiments laid the foundations for the concept of tumours possessing specific or unique antigens (Reisfeld and Cheresh 1987).

Tumour antigens are most readily demonstrable in studies in animals. Chemically induced tumours in animals express antigens unique to the carcinogen and the tumour produced, even when induced in the same animal; on occasions common antigens have been documented. Many of these tumours, in contrast to those occurring in man, are sarcomas. Virally induced tumours, on the other hand, express viral and/or virally induced antigens, which are the same on all tumours, induced by the same virus, even if arising in more than one species of animal. Unique antigens, however, have been described in virally induced tumours. Two types of antigens may be located on the tumour cell surface: (1) tumour-specific antigen (TSA), unique to the tumour cell; and (2) tumour-associated antigen (TAA)—found on both tumour and on non-malignant cells—histocompatibility (class I and II), oncofetal, differentiation, viral, and various other antigens (see Fig. 3.1).

'Spontaneous tumours' in animals and man lack readily detectable TSA, but express to a variable degree (both deletions and enhanced expression) TAA. Many tumour cells have increased expression of oncofetal antigens (e.g., carcino-embryonic antigens, CEA) and differentiation antigens, whilst the class I (HLA) antigens are reduced, altered or absent. In some tumours, e.g. melanoma, expression of HLA-II antigens have been documented and shown to be associated with a poor prognosis. Heterogeneity of antigen expression, both TSA and TAA, within a given tumour is a common finding and is thought to represent clonal selectivity, aberrations of the malignant genome and modulation of antigen expression with phases of the cell cycle (Reisfeld and Cheresh 1987).

TSA and TAA are shed readily into the circulation and are detected either as free antigen or as a complex with antibody. Increased levels of circulating oncofetal antigens (CEA, alpha-fetoprotein, prostate-specific antigen, carbohydrate-associated—CA series, etc.) in the circulation are regarded as reflecting tumour anaplasia and/or tumour cell volume. Serial serum measurements are used by clinicians to assess response to therapy and monitor recurrence (see Chapter 9, pp. 186–7). The presence of immune complexes is a reflection of the antigenicity of the shed antigen and the ability of host defences to mount a suitable humoral response. Circulating complexes are cleared from the circulation by the reticuloendothelial system. Much of the antibody response (polyclonal, monoclonal) raised against human tumour cells is directed against TAA. Difficulty in producing antibodies reactive with putative TSA, may be a reflection of absence of TSA or 'weak antigenicity' and/or inability to mount an appropriate response due to suppressor mechanisms. Recent studies in patients with cancer, e.g., melanoma, using injections of autologous or homologous irradiated tumour cells in conjunction with pre-treatment with cyclophosphamide, has resulted in the appearance of a tumour-specific humoral response. Cyclophosphamide has been shown, in animal studies, to abolish the activity of T suppressor cells.

Figure 3.1 outlines, in a schematic form, the TSA and TAA found on the surface of cancer cells and their possible relationship to humoral and cell-mediated host responses.

3.4 Anti-tumour CMI

3.4.1 Introduction

Although the presence of TSAs in most human solid cancers is still a matter of controversy, in many animal models (induced by chemical or viral carcinogens) anti-tumour CMI is well documented. In such models, the host is able to resist a tumour challenge (usually of a defined tumour volume and route of administration), following previous exposure to the same tumour or its cell components, in particular, cell membrane extracts (presumed TSA). Also, concomitant immunity is documented in many tumour-bearing animals—resistance of such an animal to challenge with the same tumour at another site. Adoptive immunity has been demonstrated in a number of cell transfer experiments in animals, using tumour cells with or without sensitized or immune lymphocytes. The presence of the latter lymphocytes, e.g., from tumour-draining lymph nodes, will inhibit the establishment of a tumour with the usual tumour-inducing innoculum of malignant cells.

In man, as well as animals, delayed type hypersensitivity (DTH) responses have been detected *in vivo* (often in the presence of a substantial residual tumour load) by injections of autologous tumour cells or tumour cell extracts intradermally. Skin-window experiments (exposure of viable autologous tumour cells to freshly produced wounds in the skin) induces an enhanced migration of lymphoreticular cells into such wounds, due to undefined chemotactic stimuli released by the tumour cells.

In vitro experiments confirm the presence of various and variable anti-tumour host defences, both in man and experimental animals. Tumour cells (and tumour cell extracts) are able to induce a blastogenic response when cultured with autologous blood or lymph node lymphocytes. Absence of reactivity of lymphocytes to co-culture with normal epithelial cells obtained from tissues of the same histological type as the tumour, suggest the presence of TSA on tumour cells. In such experiments, host lymphoreticular cells infiltrating the tumour often have been removed from the isolated tumour cell preparations. In man, it has been shown that the ability of autologous regional tumour-draining lymph node lymphocytes (particularly those from the most proximal group of nodes) to undergo such *in vitro* reactivity is reduced, compared with blood lymphocytes. Cell mixing experiments suggest that inhibition of reactivity is due to the presence of 'suppressor' T lymphocytes. The mechanism of suppression by such cells, however, is still poorly defined.

Assessment of general lymphocyte reactivity *in vitro* (e.g., ability to undergo lymphocyte transformation with a variety of polyclonal mitogens—phytohaemagglutinin, conconavalin A, and pokeweed mitogen) does reveal evidence of hyporeactivity, especially in lymphocytes from the regional tumour-draining lymph nodes. However, the activity of lymphocytes (blood and nodal), which in some cases show anergy, appears to be related to tumour load, being more pronounced in patients with extensive metastatic disease. Alterations in the ratio of $CD4^+$ to $CD8^+$ cells do occur, but do not always correlate with the hyporeactivity detected *in vitro*. The ability of such patients to mount a DTH response to topical antigens (new or recall) is substantially reduced. Many of these patients, however, are malnourished and the contribution of the latter to the cutaneous anergy and lymphocyte hyporeactivity is probably significant (see Chapter 6). Table 3.2 summarizes the CMI responses elicited in man.

3.4.2. Cytotoxic T killer cells

In man, data has accumulated from patients with severe defects of T lymphocytes—pharmacologically suppressed transplant recipients, congenitally acquired T cell defects, acquired immune deficiency syndrome (AIDS)—demonstrating the crucial role of T lymphocytes, particularly in preventing the development of malignant disease (lymphomas, cervical, and skin cancers), with a postulated viral aetiology. In rodents, thymectomy or congenital absence of the thymus, or treatment with anti-lymphocyte serum and complement, increases significantly the susceptibility of such animals to tumours induced by oncogenic viruses (polyoma, Gross leukaemia, Moloney sarcoma).

The ability of the host to mount an effective CMI response to tumours is determined by a complex array of factors: (1) the presence of TSA—the latter has to be strongly immunogenic, readily exposed on the cell surface, and be present on most, if not all, tumour cells; (2) the processing of

Table 3.2. Host CMI responses elicited in man

Nature of responses elicited/detected

In vivo

1. *DTH*
   New/recall antigens; innoculation with autologous cancer cells
2. *Skin 'Window'*
   Lymphoreticular migration—application of cancer cells to wounds
3. *Tumour lymphoreticular infiltrate*
   TIL: ↑(T, Th, Ts)
   ↓(B, NK)
   TIM: ↑MO

NB: No convincing evidence for improved survival with increased TIL/TIM, possibly the reverse

In vitro

1. *General reactivity*
   ↓Response to mitogens and alloantigens; presence of Ts cells
2. *Tumour reactivity*
   TSA detected by co-culturing autologous tumour cells and lymphocytes—blood, tumour-draining lymph nodes
3. *Killer cells*
   NK/LAK and MHC-restricted T killer cells—generated by co-culture with tumour cells and IL-2

↑, increased; ↓, decreased; T, T lymphocyte; Ts, T suppressor lymphocyte; B, B lymphocyte; MO, macrophage; Th, T helper lymphocyte; NK, natural killer cell; TIL, tumour-infiltrating lymphocyte; TIM, tumour-infiltrating macrophage; LAK, lymphokine-activated killer cell.

TSA—this involves the recognition of epitopes as foreign, by autologous T lymphocytes, requires the collaboration of *in situ* macrophages/dendritic cells for antigen processing and presentation to T cell antigen receptors in association with HLA-DR, and the release of modulator cytokines (IL-1, IL-2); (3) the generation of T helper cells and induction and proliferation of MHC-restricted (and probably MHC-non-restricted) T cytotoxic killer cells; (4) appropriate transport to sites of malignant cell proliferation and transcapillary or postcapillary venule migration into tumour cell milieu, interaction with and lytic damage of the tumour cell. Differential expression of HLA (class I antigens)—down-regulation or absence in anaplastic tumour—may be partly responsible for failure of lysis of tumour cells by cytotoxic T killer cells. Characterization of tumour-infiltrating lymphocytes (TILs) detected within progressively growing human solid tumours (the usual surgically resected specimen) reveal a significant percentage of the lymphocytes to be $CD3^+$, $CD8^+$. Functionally, however, many of the cells fail to show significant tumour specific cytotoxicity. *In vitro* culture of the TILs, however, in the presence of tumour cells and a continual source of IL-2, generates MHC-restricted and MHC-non-restricted T killer cells, to a variable degree. This suggests that inadequate secretion of cytokines, in particular IL-2, within the tumour cell milieu may be a crucial factor in the failed CMI response. Defects in either the afferent or efferent limb (or both) can result in an inadequate or deficient anti-tumour T cytolytic response (see Vanky 1986).

Figure 3.2 outlines the potential killer cell mechanisms that may be operative *in vivo* in inhibiting or abolishing tumour cell growth.

3.4.3 Natural killer (NK) cells

The absence of an increased incidence of 'spontaneous tumours' in nude mice (thymic-deficient) suggests that other non-T cell anti-tumour mechanisms may play an important role in the control of cancer. Studies in animals suggest such a role for NK cells. Nude mice are susceptible to the development of NK-resistant tumours. Similarly, strains of mice with high NK cell activity in their various lymphoreticular compartments, are less likely to sustain the growth of NK-sensitive tumour cells, compared with strains showing low levels of natural cytotoxicity. Beige mice, which lack a normal functioning natural killer cell mechanism, show a substantially reduced ability to reject tumour cell innoculums, particularly malignant cells, known to be sensitive to the action of NK cells. Numerous studies in animals have documented the role of NK cells in preventing metastatic spread of cancer cells (see Section 3.6). Suppression of NK cell activity by surgery, with its attendant enhanced circulating load of tumour cells, in several animal models have revealed enhanced tumour growth, dissemination, and diminished survival. Most recently, treatment of animals with monoclonal antibodies specific for NK cells, together with complement to lyse the cells, has been shown to facilitate tumour growth and spread.

The relevance of such studies to man, as yet, is poorly defined. NK cells show a variable distribution and activity in different lymphoid compartments, being present in significant numbers and showing activity in blood but are virtually absent from the normal thymus. Many patients bearing solid tumours, particularly where there is no clinical evidence of spread, appear to have normal NK cell activity of their circulating blood lymphocytes. NK cells are present in lymph nodes, albeit the number of such cells are less than those found in blood, but there is no evidence of modulation of NK cell activity by either the presence of metastatic deposits in the nodes or their proximity to growing solid tumours.

NK cells are found in the large granular lymphocyte (LGL) subset of cells (see Chapter 1, Section 1.5.3.) The cells are non-B, non-T, Fc (IgG) receptor-bearing lymphocytes which belong to the lymphoid lineage and

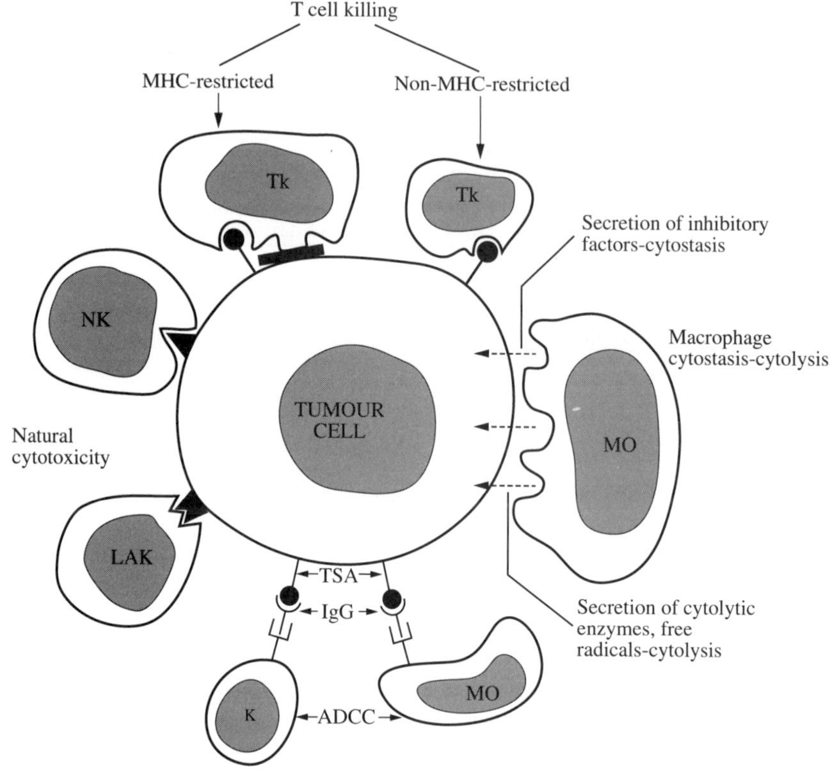

TSA, tumour specific antigen (⚲)
HLA-I, histocompatability antigens (A,B,C,) (▬)
Tk , killer lymphocyte
NK, natural killer cell (▲: glycoproteins)
LAK, lymphokine-activated killer cell (▲: glycoproteins)
K, killer cell (ADCC)
MO, macrophage
ADCC, antibody-dependent cellular cytotoxicity
IgG, immunoglobulin G (Y)

Fig. 3.2. Anti-tumour cytotoxic and cytostatic mechanisms operative *in vivo*.

may possibly arise from common pre-thymic precursors of T lymphocytes. The majority of cells express defined membrane phenotypic markers, ($CD16^+$, $CD56^+$) but overlap with other cell subsets expressing other markers ($CD2^+$, $CD8^+$, $CD3^+$). NK cells lyse syngeneic, allogeneic, and xenogeneic cells (normal, transformed or malignant). In man and animals, they appear to lyse tumour cells, without damaging normal cell types, through interaction with glycoprotein membrane moieties. Their activity is markedly enhanced by the cytokines, in particular IFN-γ. Stimulation with IL-2 leads to an expansion of the spectrum of target cells killed, as well as enhanced lytic activity (see Chapter 7). Such cells are referred to as lymphokine-activated killer (LAK) cells and are believed to be derived from the LGL subset. The efficacy of LAK cells to kill a variety of tumour cells in animals (primary and metastatic) is well documented. Their current use in clinical trials in man suggest a beneficial role in particular tumour types, e.g., melanoma and renal cell cancer. In such studies, large numbers of LAK cells and maximum doses of IL-2 are administered to patients.

The selective distribution of NK cells throughout the different lymphoreticular compartments suggests a selective migration to such sites. Investigations of solid tumours in man reveal very few, if any, NK cells within the tumour cell milieu. Precursors of LAK cells are found in solid tumours, but like NK cells, there is very little LAK cell activity detected in freshly isolated TILs. *In vitro* culture of TILs, with RIL-2, however, does generate in prolonged culture enhanced NK and LAK cell activity. Inability to generate cytokines within the tumour cell milieu or failure of entry may explain the absence of such important cytotoxic mechanisms and offer an explanation for progressive tumour growth.

3.4.4 Monocytes-macrophages

Convincing data has accumulated, predominantly from animal studies, documenting the importance of monocytes-macrophages in anti-tumour host defences. Blood monocytes from rodents bearing a variety of tumours, when mixed with such tumour cells *in vitro*, cause inhibition of tumour cell growth. Removal or inhibition of blood monocytes by pre-treatment with anti-macrophage serum and silica respectively, results in enhancement of tumour growth in certain animal tumour models. Activation, on the other hand, e.g., by pre-treatment of animals with *Corynebacterium parvum*, can result in inhibition of *in vivo* tumour growth.

Such studies are not possible in man, but there is indirect evidence confirming the relevance of the monocyte-macrophage to tumour–host interactions. Investigations in man have usually shown an enhanced activity (enhanced expression of Fc (Ig) receptors, increased intracellular enzymes) of circulating blood monocytes in patients with various solid cancers, e.g., lung, breast. Pathologists have documented, over a number of years, the presence of sinus histiocytosis in regional tumour-draining lymph nodes and its association with an improved survival in various solid cancers—breast, stomach, etc.

The majority of solid tumours in man and experimental animals show a prominent macrophage infiltrate. The tumour-infiltrating macrophages (TIMs) are often not readily discernible on routine histological assessment (due to alteration of their processes and distortion of their normal morphology), but can be readily detected by specific monoclonal antibodies directed to membrane-associated determinants. In human tumours (breast, colon, lung, etc.), the content of TIM can vary from 10 to 40 per cent. The chemotactic factors for such a mononuclear infiltrate are unknown. Although expressing Fc (Ig) and C3 receptors, normal or enhanced phagocytosis, many of the TIMs are deficient in cytolytic and other enzymes (arginase, lysozyme, α-1 anti-trypsin), and probably show defective release of free radicals. In fact, some studies suggest that TIM may produce growth-promoting factors that induce paracrine augmentation of tumour cell growth. Although there is no good correlation between the numbers of TIM and rate of tumour growth, there is some evidence in man that a high content is a poor prognostic factor.

Macrophages within tumours ingest necrotic or damaged cells, they express class II histocompatibility antigens, but their ability to process and express TSA/TAA is poorly studied. Both helper/inducer ($CD4^+$) and suppressor/cytotoxic ($CD8^+$) cells are located within tumours, but the precise interrelationship between macrophages and T cells is unclear. Macrophages are known to be activated by both non-specific macrophage-activating factors (MAF: bacteria, endotoxins, chemicals, etc.) and specific macrophage-activating factors (SMAF: secreted by activated T cells). Such activation enhances their ability to induce cytostasis as well as cytolysis. TIMs are known to secrete inhibitory factors, e.g., PGE_2 and either directly through its action on membranes or via activation of T suppressor cells can induce suppression of immune reactivity and inhibit the activity of cytotoxic T and/or NK cell activity. Monocytes-macrophages are important sources of cytokines (IL-1, TNF), which modulate immune responses, and themselves are stimulated by various cytokines (IL-2, IFN-γ, M-CSF). Very few studies, to date, have evaluated the role and interactions of these different cytokines with TIMs.

3.5 Anti-tumour humoral immunity

In many animal tumour models, a humoral anti-tumour response is elicited during tumour growth. Such a response, *per se*, is usually not adequate to abort the progressive growth of malignant clones. Anti-tumour antibodies, however, can cause damage to tumour cells *in vitro* or *in vivo* by inducing complement-mediated lysis of tumour cells coated with immunoglobulin or by an antibody-dependent cellular cytotoxicity (ADCC) mediated by K cells (see Fig. 3.2 and Section 1.5.3). The highest titre of free antibody is usually detected in the early phase of tumour growth. Interaction of tumour-specific antibody with TSA can lead to membrane redistribution and endocytosis of the immune complex by the tumour cell. This effect may be important in antigen modulation and thus leads to an ineffective anti-tumour response to TSA. This may occur either by blocking and preventing exposure of TSA to cytotoxic T cells or inducing internalization of the complex and preventing K cell activity and complement-mediated lysis. Conversely, the complex can be shed into the local milieu or the circulation. The shedding of TSA or the immune complex could result in interaction with lymphoreticular cells (via antigen) and prevent tumour cell lysis by T cells and monocytes by acting as 'blocking factors'. The role of such a 'blocking mechanism', in man, is not well documented, but excess TSAs are present in the circulation and increased substantially with progressive tumour growth in experimental tumour models in animals.

Most tumours contain a substantial amount of immunoglobulin *in situ*. The latter, however, is usually taken up cytophilically by the TIMs and appears to be non-specific Ig. Usually, very few B cells are found in most human solid tumours, and there is little evidence for *in situ* production of antibody directed against TSA. Humoral responses, on the other hand, are well documented in patients with various solid cancers. These circulating antibodies have been shown to interact with tumour cell lines as well as freshly isolated tumours cells, and the majority appear to be directed against membrane TAA or intracellular components rather than TSA. The presence of such antibodies in the circulation, however, has little bearing on the clinical progress of the disease and response to therapy.

Almost a century ago, surgeons commented on the apparent prominent lymph nodes, found adjacent to a variety of solid cancers. Such alterations in size, shape, and consistency of the tumour-draining lymph nodes was regarded as a beneficial host response. Subsequent alterations in microarchitecture, histiocytosis, prominent follicles, and germinal centres (B lymphocyte compartment) and a variable expansion of the paracortical area (T lymphocyte compartment)—were shown to be associated with increased numbers of macrophages, B lymphocytes, and T lymphocytes, respectively. The stimuli for such changes are not defined and there is no convincing evidence that they are induced by TSA. Attempts at generating homologous MABs, *in vitro*, using lymphocytes isolated from such lymph nodes have not been very successful in generating MABs directed specifically at the tumour cells, suggesting that the enhanced B lymphocyte proliferation is not directed specifically at the cancer cell.

3.6 Tumour metastasis

In the 1860s, the invasion of veins and lymphatics by viable tumour cells was documented histologically. Later, tumour cells were isolated from the venous circulation and subsequent post-mortem studies documented the presence of tumour emboli in lungs of patients who died from malignant disease. Numerous studies have detected the presence of significant numbers of tumour cells in the venous effluent from a variety of solid cancers, the numbers being enhanced substantially during anaesthesia and surgical procedures.

A century ago, Paget, based on his studies of the pattern of metastatic spread in patients with breast cancer, postulated the importance of the microenvironment in inducing the growth of entrapped tumour emboli. On the other hand, Ewing in the early part of this century, stressed the importance of the vascular architecture and the haemodynamics of the circulation. Both pathophysiological mechanisms are believed to be important in determining the organ distribution and growth of metastatic deposits (Schirmacher 1985).

Host defence mechanisms are thought to play a crucial role at three anatomical sites: (1) the site of primary tumour cell growth and local haemolymphatic invasion; (2) the haemolymphatic compartments (vascular and lymphatic), including the 'filter' role of lymph nodes; and (3) the *in situ* lymphoreticular defences within individual organs of tumour cell arrest—liver, lungs, bone marrow, etc.

Rapid cell proliferation is believed to be linked to alterations in the genome, with resultant chromosomal alterations, enhanced and/or inappropriate expression of various proto-oncogenes and their secreted products, increased production of growth factors and augmentation of their membrane receptors, resulting in increased mitogenicity and autocrine-driven cell growth, and cell replication. These metabolic abnormalities, as well as structural and functional changes in the cell membrane (e.g., modulation of expression of adhesion molecules and surface lectins) lead to enhanced tumour cell aggressiveness, loss of contact inhibition, and to local invasion. The latter is associated with an increased adhesion of the malignant cell to the basement membrane through laminin and other adhesive receptors and the increased release of various proteolytic enzymes causing breakdown of sub-epithelial collagen and alteration of surrounding ground substance. The acquisition of a tumour vasculature, induced by angiogenesis factors secreted by the malignant cells, is crucial to the delivery of oxygen and essential nutrients to the rapidly expanding mass of neoplastic cells. Also, it is an important route for the eventual entry by invading tumour cells and their subsequent dissemination. (Table 3.3)

An important route of tumour cell dissemination is via the regional tumour-draining lymphatic channels and lymph nodes. The tumour-draining lymph nodes, in particular adjacent to the solid growth, undergo macro- and micro-architectural alterations suggestive of altered immune responses to filtered tumour cells and/or cellular products (e.g., membrane antigens). Although lymph nodes have been shown, in some animal models, to inhibit tumour cell dissemination, in others, their ability to function as a 'mechanical filter' has been shown to be inefficient. Transmigration of lymph nodes, even by large tumour cells, is well documented; the tumour

Table 3.3. Tumour cell factors inducing metastatic invasion

Mechanism	Factors underlying mechanism
Growth Proliferation	1. ↑ Oncogene activation and secretion of gene products 2. ↑ Growth factor receptor expression and secretion of growth factors
Local spread	1. ↓ Membrane adhesion molecules/lectins 2. ↑ Secretion of proteolytic enzymes and destruction of ground substance and stromal elements
Invasion of blood and lymphatic vessels	1. Direct entry as well as through wide vessel pores in the capillary-lymphatic cell wall 2. Fibrin coating of tumour emboli affords protection against kinetic forces in blood and anti-tumour CMI

cells eventually reaching the venous system via the thoracic duct. Also, venous–lymphatic communications have been demonstrated within lymph nodes of some species and are thought to represent a further possible site of entry of malignant cells into the vascular compartment.

The presence of metastatic deposits within regional lymph nodes is a poor prognostic feature and is a biological indication of more distal dissemination. Surgical removal of such involved nodes reduces the risk of local recurrence but probably does not influence overall survival. Conversely, removal of uninvolved lymph nodes (even where they have undergone hyperplastic changes) does not appear to compromise patient survival.

Very few, probably less than 1 per cent, of the tumour cells that enter the venous circulation survive transport to distant organs. The mechanical stresses imparted on the tumour emboli by the blood flow are mainly responsible for this death rate. Coating of tumour aggregates with fibrin and platelets probably provides protection from both the stresses of blood flow as well as host defence mechanisms. Although the evidence in man is inconclusive, substantial data has accumulated from a variety of animal studies that NK cells play a crucial role in preventing the establishment of tumour metastases. The latter studies suggest that NK cells are most effective in dealing with circulating tumour cells, especially in the early phase of tumour dissemination. Once metastatic disease is established, NK cells appear to be less efficacious as anti-tumour agents.

As mentioned previously, the 'soil' probably plays a crucial role in the establishment and progressive growth of tumour emboli. Paradoxically, many of the common sites of tumour metastatic growth—lungs, liver, lymph nodes, skeletal system—are rich in lymphoreticular cells. Induction of suppressor mechanisms by tumour cell products (release of PGE_2) and possible enhancement of tumour cell growth by molecules released by tissue macrophages, have all been invoked to offer an explanation. The precise mechanisms, however, have not been delineated.

3.7 Summary

Substantial evidence is available from both animal experiments and clinical data from man, that the host is able (and often does) generate an anti-tumour immune response. Prolonged inability to generate an effective host response can lead to the development of tumours, particularly those induced by DNA oncoviruses. The anti-tumour response, particularly in man, is obviously inadequate to prevent tumour growth in cancer-bearing patients. Both a humoral and CMI response can be determined, to a variable degree. Various factors—failure of reactivity to TSA (in contrast to TAA), inhibition of immune reactivity by suppressor mechanisms, secretion of tumour-growth promoting factors by lymphoreticular cells (e.g., TIMs), inadequate release of cytokines within tumour cell milieu, etc.—may all contribute to progressive tumour growth and dissemination. Major advances in our understanding of basic biological mechanisms (e.g., oncogenes and gene control mechanisms, growth factors, and cytokines), as well as the introduction of immune biological modifiers (IL-2, IFN, TNF) into clinical practice, should improve our understanding of the cancer process and the anti-tumour role of host immune defences.

References and further reading

Schirmacher, V. (1985). Cancer metastasis: Experimental approaches, theoretical concepts and impacts for treatment strategies. *Advances in cancer research*, **43**, 1–73.

Vanky, F. (1986). Membrane structures involved in auto-tumour recognition. *Biochemia Biophsica Acta*, **865**, 253–65.

Reisfeld, R.A. and Cheresh, D.A. (1987). Human tumour antigens. *Advances in Immunology*, **40**, 323–77.

4

Trauma and the immune response

H.C. Polk Jr. and W. Cheadle

4.1 Introduction

Trauma is an immense, world-wide, socio-economic problem that predominantly affects young people. In the United States, it is the leading cause of death in those under 45 years of age and the resultant morbidity often leads to significant disability. The cost in terms of hospital care, loss of productivity, and emotional stress is staggering. Efforts directed at accident prevention and efficient triage, and to the establishment of properly staffed trauma centres are of paramount importance. Should the badly injured patient survive a serious head injury and/or major haemorrhage, the next threat to life will be infection. Sepsis has been recognized as the most common cause of late death in these patients and accounts for much of the morbidity in those who recover from infection. The reasons why injured patients are at such risk of infection are discussed in this chapter.

The relationship between the nervous and the immune system following trauma is poorly understood and under investigation. Recent reviews have highlighted the complex nature of the tremendous surge of hormone and catecholamine output from the pituitary-adrenal axis following trauma, which may be mediated through the spinal cord along afferent neurons from the site of tissue destruction. Also, an immediate and generalized depression of the immune system exists, and this continues to be an ongoing area of research interest.

Virtually all components of the immune response have been found to be depressed following injury including macrophage, lymphocyte, and neutrophil function; delayed type hypersensitivity (DTH) responses, immunoglobulin (Ig) and interferon (IFN) production, and serum opsonic capacity. Serum peptides, which suppress lymphocyte proliferation *in vitro*, have been defined, and the immunosuppressive role of excessive complement activation has also been recognized. Immune failure occurs early after trauma and the rapidity with which immune function returns to normal may be the best indicator of clinical recovery. Indeed, immediate down-regulation of the immune response may be a protective mechanism for the host, lest too vigorous an early host response creates a catabolic situation incompatible with early survival. (Polk *et al.* 1986)

4.2 The immune system

Cells, opsonins, and mediators make up the immune system. Its role in host defence has been conceptualized as having specific and non-specific participants and schematicized as encounter, recognition, activation, deployment, discrimination, and regulation (see Chapter 1). Non-specific factors include mechanical barriers, such as the skin and gastrointestinal tract, complement components, inflammatory mediators, cytokines, and the process of phagocytosis itself. These are directed against all foreign antigens whether or not the host has been previously challenged by a particular microbial organism.

4.2.1 The non-specific system

The complement cascade is a series of enzymatic cleavage reactions that are triggered by either antigen-antibody complexes (classical pathway) or bacterial cell wall components (alternate pathway), and must occur in sequential fashion to be effective. The latter pathway does not require prior immunization for activation and thus represents a mechanism for immediate defence against any foreign antigen. Some of the cleavage products are capable of direct bacterial lysis, and activated complement anaphylatoxin components (C3a and C5a) act with kinins and fibrin degradation products to increase capillary permeability by causing histamine release. Complement components are capable of recruiting neutrophils by chemotactic action, and facilitate both phagocytosis and bacterial killing through opsonization of bacteria and stimulation of neutrophil degranulation.

Histamine, kinins, and arachidonic acid metabolites are involved as soluble mediators in both the inflammatory and immune responses. Tissue injury results in the release of histamine from mast cells, as well as bradykinin and kallikrin production. These substances act directly on vascular endothelium to increase permeability with production of local oedema and accumulation of cellular and protein elements of the immune system at the site of injury. Arachidonic acid is produced by breakdown of cellular membranes and the action of phospholipase A. Arachidonic acid is, in turn, broken down by either lipo-oxygenase to form leukotrienes or cyclo-oxygenase to form prostaglandins (PGs) and thromboxanes. These eicosanoids have various effects that mediate the inflammatory process. For example, PGs inhibit platelet aggregation while thromboxanes promote such aggregation. Most of the inflammatory mediators are formed quickly and act locally where their effect is maximum and short lived because of rapid metabolism.

The process of phagocytosis is essential for the eradication of most invading microorganisms, and is carried out primarily by neutrophils and tissue macrophages. This multi-step process includes adherence of the phagocytic cells to capillary endothelium, migration to the site of inflammation via chemotaxis, opsonization of the foreign material (mostly by complement and/or Igs), engulfment of the organisms into the cell, and finally microbial killing and degradation. Disorders of phagocytosis are all associated with an increased risk of infection and span the spectrum from low neutrophil production to defective degranulation and intracellular killing.

Cytokines are peptide hormones that allow cells to communicate between themselves. There are at least eight interleukins (ILs) now recognized, but IL-1 and IL-2 have been studied most extensively. Although part of the non-specific system, they are produced by cells of the immune system in response to antigenic stimulation. Tumour necrosis factor alpha (TNF-α) may well be one of the final common mediators of the overall inflammatory response as it shares many of the properties of IL-1. IFN-γ is produced primarily by mononuclear cells and has been shown to increase class II histocompatibility antigens (HLA-DR) on the surface of monocytes-macrophages which may amplify foreign antigen recognition.

4.2.2 The specific immune system

The specific immune system includes B and T lymphocytes, and antigen-presenting (accessory) cells (APCs), such as macrophages (see Chapter 1, Section 1.3.) The initial step in the specific immune response involves foreign antigen recognition, uptake, degradation, and expression on the cell surface of the macrophage. IL-1 is produced, and T helper cells bind to the foreign antigen in contiguity with HLA-DR on the macrophage cell surface. The activated T helper cell (CD4$^+$) then produces IL-2, which, in turn, stimulates B cell maturation into plasma cells that subsequently produce antibody. Such antibodies are specific to the original foreign antigen, and memory B cells are then capable of an augmented, rapid secondary response to previously recognized antigen. T suppressor cells (CD8$^+$) may also be activated by the initial process, particularly if PGE$_2$ is released by macrophages, and these suppressor lymphocytes inhibit their $CD4^+$ counterparts. Many of the non-specific participants, such as the cytokines, inflammatory mediators, and the process of phagocytosis itself, are often dependent upon the specific components as well. For example, phagocytosis is much more efficient for opsonized antigens, and in general, specific participants amplify the non-specific response.

4.3 Immune failure

The multi-system organ failure syndrome was first described at the same time that depressed cell-mediated immunity (CMI), in the form of anergic delayed type hypersensitivity (DTH) skin testing, was noted in severely ill patients. Patients classified as anergic or hyporeactive were said to have an increased risk of infection and death. Curiously, patients may remain anergic for weeks after recovery from infection or trauma. Over 90 per cent of severely injured patients are often anergic on admission to the hospital and the duration of anergy increases both with the severity of injury and the development of major infection. The development of monoclonal antibodies (MABs) and more sophisticated assays of specific immunological function has led to the discovery of a variety of defects associated with trauma, sepsis, and multi-system organ failure. Infection has been present in half or more of the patients who have concomitant multi-system organ failure; most of the information available pertaining to immune failure has come from patients with severe infection or following injury.

4.4 Cell-mediated immunity (CMI)

A variable and, as yet, inadequately defined inhibition of CMI is present in the severely injured and/or septic patient. The following cellular host defences have been investigated and found to play a role (Polk *et al.* 1986).

4.4.1 Monocytes

Major trauma significantly alters the composition and function of monocytes-macrophages, lymphocytes, and neutrophils. There is a relative monocytosis after severe injury, the monocytes increasing from 10 per cent to over 30 per cent, one week after injury. Also, we have found a monocytosis that peaked on the eleventh day in hospital following trauma and only slowly returned to normal over several weeks. The surface expression of the class II HLA-DR on peripheral blood monocytes was measured in 60 patients and was depressed in most, immediately following severe trauma and during sepsis.

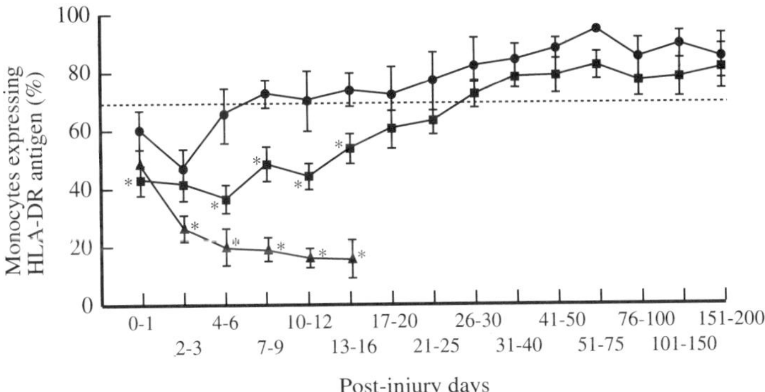

Fig. 4.1. The percentage of monocytes that expressed HLA-DR antigen over the patient's hospital course. ●, uneventful recovery; ■, major infection; ▲, dead; *, denotes significantly different from uneventful recovery group;, - - - -, lower limits of the normal range. (From Cheadle and Polk, reproduced by permission).

However, when the patients were grouped according to clinical outcome (uneventful recovery, major infection, and death) an interesting pattern arose (Fig. 4.1). The percentage of monocytes that expressed the HLA-DR antigen returned to the normal range by one week in the first group, by three weeks in those with major infection, but never in those who eventually died. Thus, antigen expression served as a useful marker, or predictor, of clinical outcome in such patients. When monocytes were incubated with bacterial lipopolysaccharide (LPS), those patients who survived had enhanced HLA-DR antigen expression (stimulated towards the normal range), while monocytes from patients who died were relatively resistant to stimulation. As LPS is thought to externalize all preformed antigen to the cell surface, an 'exhaustion' of HLA-DR antigen in the patients who died with an accompanying inability to synthesize new antigen is a possibility. Expression of HLA-DR antigen may correlate with the ability of these cells to present foreign antigen and thus initiate a specific immune response.

Monocyte HLA-DR expression within 24 hours of hospital admission, assessment of bacterial contamination, age, and injury severity, have been combined to formulate a useful outcome predictive score (OPS). The injury severity score (ISS) is adjusted for the patient's age and the result expressed as per cent LD_{50}. Results are multiplied by simple scaling factors for degree of contamination and monocyte HLA-DR expression. This is the first trauma scoring system to include a valid assessment of host defence processes, and to successfully identify (Fig. 4.2) those patients who eventually developed major infection and subsequently died from sepsis. Interestingly, the presence of hypotension and the amount of blood transfused did not

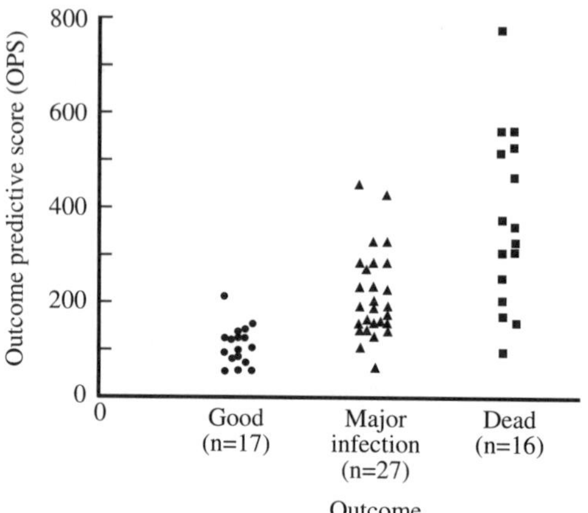

Fig. 4.2. Scattergram of the outcome predictive score (OPS) according to clinical outcome groups. A score of more than 150 was highly predictive of major infection or death. (From Cheadle *et al.* 1989*b*, reproduced by permission).

correlate with the development of infection and multi-system organ failure; HLA-DR antigen expression was the best discriminator of poor clinical outcome (Livingston *et al.* 1988).

4.4.2 Lymphocytes

Abnormalities in lymphocytes were first documented as depressed blastogenesis to mitogenic stimulation following surgery. Later, such changes were noted following injury and infection, particularly in patients who had sustained burns. Most studies have shown a decrease in the helper/suppressor lymphocyte ratio that is due primarily to a reduction in helper cells. These results complemented the initial observations of excessive suppressor cell activity (determined *in vitro* by the mixed lymphocyte reaction—(MLR)) from severely burned patients. Increased T suppressor cell activity has been shown in this setting and defective T cell IL-2 and Ia surface receptor expression has been found in mice subjected to thermal injury.

Our study population of 60 severely injured patients was analysed for several functional lymphocyte subsets. A nadir in the total peripheral lymphocyte count occurred between days 2 and 4 post-injury, with a gradual return towards the normal range throughout the hospital course, but there was no correlation with eventual clinical outcome in these patients. Initial reduction in total blood lymphocytes, has also been seen after operation alone. Reduction in both T helper and T suppressor cells was seen with gradual return to normal as well. Of note, the helper:suppressor ratio in patients who died was significantly greater than in survivors, at all time points measured over the first 12 days of study. In patients who died, the mean helper:suppressor ratio varied between 2.5 and 3.7. HLA-DR antigen expression was also measured on both T helper and T suppressor cells; this remained low in those patients who died, but rose to normal values in surviving patients on day 4 after injury. Natural killer cells remained low in all patients until four to five weeks into their hospital stay. The number of B cells remained unchanged in all patients throughout the study period. At this time, the precise role of T lymphocytes in the immune failure following trauma remains unclear.

4.4.3 Neutrophils

Defects of neutrophil function have been difficult to demonstrate consistently, even though their role is of paramount importance to host defences. Defective adherence and chemotaxis of leucocytes *in vitro* has been demonstrated in anergic surgical patients who became infected. Abnormalities in *in vitro* neutrophil migration have also been seen after injury, and reduction in complement-mediated chemotaxis was found in severely injured and septic patients, possibly due to membrane receptor saturation. Phagocytic capacity and intracellular killing are depressed following injury, but some workers have shown that depressed neutrophil chemiluminescence was dependent on exposure to the patient's serum. Neutrophil oxygen consumption, superoxide, and hydrogen peroxide production, all measures of intrinsic metabolic function, have been found to be depressed in severely burned patients. We were unable, however, to find a correlation between neutrophil oxidative burst, measured by flow cytometry, and patient outcome after injury.

4.5 Humoral immunity

4.5.1 Immunoglobulins

Humoral factors appear to contribute significantly to the determination of clinical outcome in injured patients. Both total serum immunoglobulins, as well as antibodies to specific bacteria from our cohort of trauma patients, were examined. Reduction of serum IgA, IgG, and IgM classes were seen immediately following injury. IgG and IgM levels remained low in patients who had undergone splenectomy and in those who had sepsis following thermal injuries. In contrast, infected patients without burns and who had not undergone splenectomy were able to increase their serum IgG and IgM levels into the normal range. These levels were significantly greater than those monitored in the group of patients who had recovered without major infection. Serum IgG levels were actually substantially increased in this group by two weeks after injury (Fig. 4.3). Thus, the non-specific

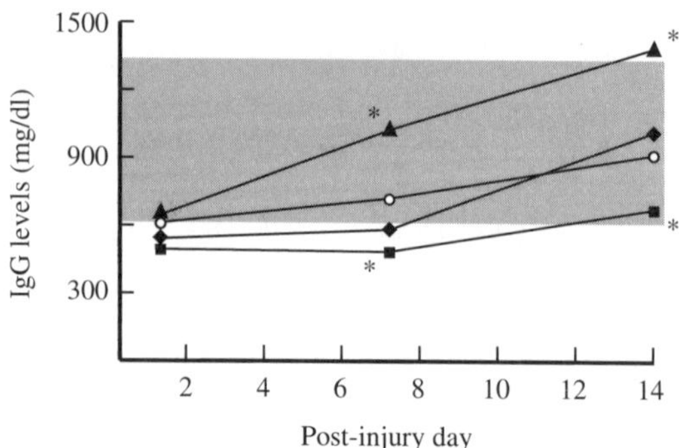

Fig. 4.3. Serial IgG levels in severely injured patients. ○, uneventful recovery; ▲, infected non-thermal; ■, infected burns; ◆, splenectomy; *, significantly different from uneventful recovery group. (From Hershman *et al.* 1988*a*, reproduced by permission).

immunoglobulin response appeared to depend on the type of injury, presence of infection, residual splenic function, and the immunoglobulin classes documented. Ability to generate high levels of IgG and IgM following injury was beneficial, particularly after splenectomy.

These patients were also examined for antibody response to *Staphylococcus aureus, Pseudomonas aeruginosa* (three separate strains), and *Escherichia coli* using an enzyme-linked immunosorbent assay (ELISA) technique (see Chapter 9, Section 9.2.3). The IgM response to *Staphylococcus aureus* was highly specific (92 per cent) but not seen in three of 10 patients with staphylococcal infections. However, two of these three died of infection and one developed a severe chronic infection, so an appropriate specific IgM response, when challenged, appeared important.

Twenty-two of 27 patients mounted antibody reponses to the Gram-negative organisms described and two patterns of response were found to be clinically relevant. These were an IgG response to *Escherichia coli*. Major infection in these patients was related to both the degree of bacterial contamination at the time of injury and the subsequent antibody responses elicited. Most patients without contamination did not mount an antibody response or become infected, but seven of eight patients with heavy contamination became infected regardless of the antibody response elicited. Six of eight patients with moderate bacterial contamination mounted a response as described to all four organisms, but only one became infected. Specific antibody responses were seen, despite anergic skin test responses, and appeared most beneficial in those with moderate bacterial contamination at injury.

4.5.2 Complement components

A decrease in circulating, stable complement components (C1, C3–5) has been shown following trauma and in patients with multi-system organ failure. Also, massive complement activation has been associated with septic shock. It has been difficult to predict the clinical outcome based on complement changes detected early in the course of trauma; many of the changes monitored may be secondary to perpetuation of the infective process.

4.5.3 Opsonins

Complement, antibodies, fibronectin, and probably other proteins, all contribute to the opsonic capacity of serum. Heat-killed, dye-stained bacteria were incubated with both pooled human serum and patient serum at four different dilutions to allow opsonization to occur. The opsonized bacteria were then incubated with single donor volunteer neutrophils and the fluorescence emitted from the ingested bacteria was measured to quantify the number that had undergone phagocytosis. Parallel samples, heated to 56°C to inactivate complement, were also measured.

Our study showed a significant reduction in the mean serum opsonic capacity in those who died compared with survivors in both total and heat-inactivated samples, as expressed by mean fluorescence intensity (Table 4.1). Such differences became most clear at the highest dilution of serum (0.5 per cent) and occurred within 24 hours of hospital admission. A *super* serum response over time was seen in four of seven patients who survived major

Table 4.1. Opsonic capacity expressed as per cent mean fluorescence for both total and heat-inactivated serum*

Complement-dependent			**Complement-independent**		
Serum conc. (%)	**Septic** (n = 21)	**Dead** (n = 9)	**Serum conc. (%)**	**Septic** (n = 21)	**Dead** (n = 8)
0.5	99.0 ± 9.0	61.0 ± 5.7	0.5	99.0 ± 7.4	58.1 ± 11.9
1.0	89.8 ± 6.4	66.0 ± 6.8	1.0	87.0 ± 5.7	53.1 ± 7.4
5.0	90.8 ± 6.1	56.7 ± 7.7	5.0	86.4 ± 4.9	54.9 ± 19.4
10.0	85.1 ± 5.9	68.0 ± 10.5	10.0	97.3 ± 7.1	66.1 ± 8.3

* From Polk *et al.* 1988, reproduced by permission.
Heat-killed, dye-stained bacteria incubated with patients' serum at various dilutions to allow opsonization to occur. Opsonized bacteria incubated with control neutrophils. Emitted fluorescence measured and used to quantify bacterial phagocytosis and thus opsonic capacity of serum.

infection, but not in the seven patients who died. This super serum response was characterized by mean fluorescence intensity values greater than 150 per cent of pooled human serum. One patient developed a consumptive opsoninopathy with chronic major infection. The ability of patient's serum to support neutrophil phagocytosis was found to be an independent predictor of clinical outcome from infection. Further, the ability to increase serum opsonic capacity in the presence of major infection proved to be beneficial to the host (Polk *et al.* 1988).

4.5.4 Cytokines

IL-1, IL-2, IFN-γ, tumour necrosis factor alpha (TNF-α), and the PGs are inflammatory mediators and cytokines that recently have been implicated in the pathophysiology of multi-system organ failure and sepsis. Following major injury, increased production of PGE_2 from inhibitory macrophages with concomitant reduction in the secretion of IL-1 has been demonstrated. We have confirmed this finding, showing that in our traumatized patients, their endogenous IFN production was low. Also, it has been shown by others that IL-2 production is suppressed in severely traumatized patients and that this suppression is dependent on the production of PGE_2. IFN production is essential for sustained macrophage participation in the cell surface interaction with T helper cells and thus critical to the generation of the specific immune response. Class II HLA antigen expression on mononuclear cells is induced by IFN and hence amplifies this specific immune response. TNF appears to be one of the final soluble mediators of inflammation, particularly when induced by endotoxin. Some studies, however, have shown a reduction in mortality in the mouse, from both bacterial infections and endotoxin shock, after TNF treatment.

4.6 Immune modulation

Freund's complete adjuvant (FCA), which induces both an enhanced antibody and DTH response to an antigen when combined with that particular antigen, initiated modern immune enhancement. Severe side-effects were associated with the use of this emulsion and spurred development of other adjuvants, using both whole bacteria (BCG—bacille Calmette-Guérin, *Corynebacterium parvum*) and cell wall products—phospholipid, lipopolysaccharide (LPS), glucan. Although fewer side-effects were noted with these preparations, timing and dosage were critical, and a narrow therapeutic window existed outside of which toxicity or even immunosuppression occurred.

Other synthetic compounds and peptides have also been studied in experimental models. Levamisole, developed as an anti-helmintic drug, has been shown to augment phagocytosis and has been critically studied in humans.

Significantly, fewer infectious complications were found in a group of anergic patients who received levamisole compared with placebo, and improved neutrophil chemotaxis and skin test reactivity was seen. Pyran, a synthetic copolymer, and avridine, a lipoidal amine, are both capable of inducing IFN production and, therefore, may be potentially useful following severe injury. Purification and synthesis of the six amino acid peptidoglycan, *N*-acetyl muramyl-L-alanyl-D-glutamine (muramyl dipeptide or MDP) resulted in efforts to isolate the active fraction of the mycobacterial cell wall. Isomers have been synthesized which are devoid of side-effects, including fever, and the therapeutic window is surprisingly wide. MDP's mode of action is thought to be through enhanced macrophage function, although B and T lymphocytes may be directly affected as well. We have pursued non-specific stimulation of the host defence response with this immunomodulator in a variety of experimental animal models in our laboratory.

4.6.1 Muramyl dipeptide

An initial model of surgical wound infection, using a *Klebsiella*-laden suture placed into the thigh adductor muscles of the mouse, confirmed the safety of MDP and demonstrated its efficacy. Mice receiving a reduced intake of food, with increased early survival following MDP pre-treatment, had reduced levels of bacteria both locally and in the blood. This effect was found to be additive to antibiotics. MDP also increased the reticulo-endothelial phagocytic index and corrected its reduction during hypo-volaemia. The incidence of anaerobic and polymicrobial abscess formation was increased when MDP was used in an experimental model of peritonitis (Cheadle *et al.* 1989*a*). However, a reduced mortality was demonstrated in both this and another model (caecal ligation and puncture). The increased abscess formation was thought to be due to an enhanced bacterial localization at the site of innoculation, because MDP has been most effective when administered 24 hours before innoculation. Its primary use in humans has been as an adjuvant to vaccines and few, if any, trials of its non-specific host stimulatory properties have been undertaken.

4.6.2 Cytokines

In addition to MDP, we have observed that LPS and IFN also restore depressed HLA-DR antigen expression in human peripheral blood monocytes following trauma. Attention has focused on the cytokines IFN and TNF as these compounds have substantial immunoregulatory potential as therapeutic agents after bacterial challenge. The optimum dosage of the recombinant murine IFN was determined to be 7500 units per day, and improvement in survival was seen when it was used both prophylactically

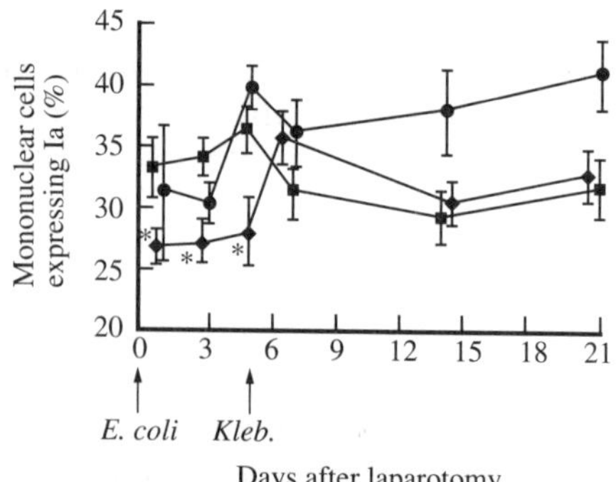

Fig. 4.4. Effect of IFN-γ treatment in the dual infection laparotomy model on the expression of Ia antigen on peripheral mononuclear cells. ■, control; ◆, *E. coli*, laparotomy and *K. pneumoniae (Kleb.)*; ●, *E. coli*, laparotomy, *K. pneumoniae*, and IFN-γ treatment; *, statistically significant different from group control ($p < 0.05$). Bars represent standard error of the mean. (From Hershman *et al.* 1988*b*, reproduced by permission).

and therapeutically in an intramuscular *Klebsiella* challenge model (see above). IFN significantly lowered the bacterial counts in the blood, and was associated with increased survival in the 'thigh suture' model.

In another model, mice underwent laparotomy with intraperitoneal innoculation of *Escherichia coli*, followed five days later by intramuscular injection of *Klebsiella pneumoniae*. Mononuclear cell Ia antigen expression was measured and was found to be significantly reduced for three days following the laparotomy. This reduction, which was associated with an increased mortality, was not seen in IFN-treated animals (Fig. 4.4). The effect of TNF has been examined in these models and similar results have been obtained, but the dosage of TNF used is very critical. Enhanced survival, with both pre-treatment and active therapy against bacterial challenge, was seen at an optimal dose of 7500 units daily. Synergy between these two cytokines has been demonstrated in humans where it has been found to enhance receptor expression on polymorphonuclear leucocytes.

4.6.3 Other biological modifiers

Immunomodulation, including specific active and passive immunization and non-specific passive immunotherapy with agents, such as granulocyte transfusions and antibody components, have been studied clinically. Plasmapheresis has been performed in patients with burns and immunization, carried out against common LPS core antigens shared by the *Enterobacteriaceae*. These have had some success, in a small number of clinical settings, but have not achieved broad clinical recognition or application. Trials currently in progress are designed to determine the efficacy of immunomodulators, such as glucan, thiotepa, and IFN, following major trauma. (Faist *et al.* 1986)

4.7 Future directions

Failure of host defences following trauma is indeed multi-factorial and complex. Various studies have demonstrated the following important defects: depressed monocyte HLA-DR expression and serum opsonic capacity; reduced endogenous IFN and IL-2 production; and increased PGE_2 production. However, trials have been slow to be introduced into clinical practice, despite identification of such defects in man and animals, and extensive laboratory work with immunomodulation both *in vitro* and in the experimental animal. Defining patients at very high risk of infection and multi-system organ failure *before* either develop, is paramount to the introduction and interpretation of clinical trials in this area. The outcome predictive score (OPS) may help in the early identification of high-risk patients.

The most promising development for traumatized patients is probably the specific immune modulation of host defences before infection, and its attendant complications arise and become established. We believe that immune enhancement, possibly with combination therapy, will become a principle treatment regimen for these patients in the future. Specific modulators and their appropriate sequence of use remain important subjects for research.

References

Cheadle, W.G., Hershman, M., Mays, B., Melton, L., and Polk, H.C., Jr. (1989*a*). Enhancement of survival from murine polymicrobial peritonitis with increased abdominal abscess formation. *Journal of Surgical Research*, **47**, 120–3.

Faist, E. *et al.* (1986). Depression of cellular immunity after major injury. Its association with posttraumatic complications and its reversal with immunomodulation. *Archives of Surgery*, **121**, 1000–1005.

Livingston, D.H., Appel, S.H., Wellhausen, S.R., Sonnenfeld, G., and Polk, H.C., Jr. (1988). Depressed interferon gamma production and monocyte HLA-DR expression after severe injury. *Archives of Surgery*, **123**, 1309–12.

Polk, H.C., Jr. *et al.* (1986). A systematic study of host defense processes in badly injured patients. *Annals of Surgery*, **204**, 282–99.

Polk, H.C. Jr., George, C.D., Hershman, M.J., Wellhausen, S.R., and Cheadle, W.G. (1988). The capacity of serum to support neutrophil phagocytosis is a vital host defence mechanism in severely injured patients. *Annals of Surgery*, **207**, 686–92.

Further reading

Cheadle, W.G. and Polk, H.C. Jr. (1991). Immune failure and modulation. In *Multiple organ failure: Pathogenesis and management* (ed. D.E. Fry). Year Book Medical Publishers, Chicago.

Cheadle, W.G., *et al.* (1989*b*). Comparison of trauma assessment scores and their use in prediction of infection and death. *Annals of Surgery*, **109**, 541–6.

Hershman, M.J., *et al.* (1988*a*). The response of immunoglobulins to infection after thermal and non-thermal injury. *Annals of Surgery*, **54**, 408–11.

Hershman, M.J., *et al.* (1988*b*). Modulation of infection by gamma interferon treatment following trauma. *Infection and Immunity*, **56**, 2412–16.

5
Sepsis and the immune response

R. Dionigi and L. Dominioni

5.1 Infection and sepsis: introduction

In spite of advances in the methods for early detection of infections and in the treatment of complications arising from infections, mortality from severe surgical sepsis remains very high. Extensive studies on the immunological status of surgical patients have shown that the susceptibility to post-operative infections is influenced not only by contamination through the operative field, but also by peri-operative impairment of immunity. The surgical patient, therefore, must be considered at risk of developing infections because of the increased ease and frequency of invasion by pathogenic microorganisms, and because containment and resolution of infectious episodes in surgery depend on the efficiency of host defence mechanisms.

5.1.1 Immunocompetence and infections in surgery

Host defences play an obvious role in infections and it has been well documented that the various components of the immune response are important in obtaining control of and inducing the resolution of infectious episodes in surgical practice. Many studies have shown that the immune factors essential for resistance to bacterial pathogens include humoral and cell-mediated immunity, neutrophils and cells of the reticuloendothelial system, and a large number of biological mediators of inflammation and the immune response.

Pre-operative

Alterations of immunocompetence may occur in the surgical patient pre-operatively, mainly as a consequence of the underlying surgical disease, such as cancer, severe malnutrition, burns, trauma or shock. Occasionally, pre-operative immunodepression is iatrogenic, being related to the administration of chemotherapeutic or immunosuppressive drugs, or to pre-operative radiotherapy (see Chapter 7). Rarely, surgical patients may have primary defects of cellular or humoral immunity. Regardless of the cause, pre-operative immunodepression is well documented to predispose patients to increased risk of developing infections following surgery.

Post-operative

Post-operative immunodepression occurs very frequently. It is well established that surgical procedures, which are carried out under general anaesthesia with significant tissue manipulation and trauma, are accompanied by a transient state of immunodepression (see Chapter, 7 Section 7.2). The cause of post-operative immunodepression has been attributed to several factors, among which the following have been identified:

(1) anaesthetic drugs;
(2) peri-operative administration of blood components;
(3) release of acute phase proteins with immunosuppressive effects;
(4) humoral mediators induced by sepsis; and
(5) immunosuppressive factors released by the surgically induced wound.

Not infrequently, surgical patients are immunocompromised as a result of the combined effects of the pre- and post-operative immunosuppressive factors listed above. Splenectomy is an operation that especially adds to the risk of post-operative infection, particularly in infants and children due to the loss of splenic defence mechanisms in combating certain infections (e.g., due to pneumococcal organisms).

5.1.2 Infection and the septic state

During the last two decades, the mechanism of immune responses to infection has been extensively investigated. It has been established that minor infections are characterized by moderate alterations of general homeostatic mechanisms, with easy control of the microbial invasion by host defences.

Conversely, severe infections, due either to overwhelming bacterial contamination, and/or to defective immune defences, are accompanied by complex changes in homeostasis. These modifications are defined as the *septic response*, and may progress in a graded fashion towards multiple organ failure (MOF), and ultimately to death.

The septic state is now recognized as a clinical syndrome, to be distinguished from microbial infection *per se*. The clinical syndrome of *sepsis* can be defined as the complex reaction of various organs and systems to microbial invasion. It is now established that the septic state may continue even after bacterial invasion is no longer demonstrable. Although linked by a cause–effect relationship, bacterial invasion and septic response are currently being investigated as two separate pathological entities. From the practical therapeutic standpoint, however, it is important to realize that in most instances control of bacterial infections may be achieved whereas it is much more difficult to control septic responses.

5.1.3 The septic response

The clinical syndrome of sepsis is characterized by a complex series of responses by various organs and systems to infection. The pathological alterations and the homeostatic modifications taking place, as a result of microbial invasion, can be categorized as: (1) local effects on infected tissues/organs; (2) acute phase responses; and (3) secondary effects on target organs/systems, distant from the site of microbial invasion.

The well-known *local effects* of sepsis are characterized by the production of exudate and by tissue necrosis in the infected site. The resulting tissue damage and impaired function of the infected organs can be quantified by scoring systems, which have been developed in recent years to assess the severity of septic responses (Dominioni *et al.* 1987).

The *acute phase responses* to microbial invasion, which have been postulated to represent defence reactions important for survival, include numerous hormonal, metabolic, haemodynamic, and immunological reactions (see Table 5.1).

The hormonal response to infections is characterized by increased release of pituitary and 'stress hormones'. These hormonal changes in turn mediate complex metabolic responses, including increased metabolic rate, increased oxygen consumption, increased gluconeogenesis, increased glucose oxidation, utilization of endogenous fat, enhanced protein turnover, fluid retention, and electrolyte imbalances.

The acute phase haemodynamic responses to severe infections are initially characterized by a hyperdynamic state with tachycardia and increased cardiac index and reduced vascular resistance, and are accompanied by increased vascular permeability. Subsequently, a low-flow state develops,

Table 5.1. Acute phase responses to infection

Metabolic/hormonal
Increased metabolic rate
Fever
Increased oxygen consumption
Increased gluconeogenesis
Reduced glucose oxidation
Insulin-resistant hyperglycaemia
Increased utilization of endogenous fat
Increased protein synthesis and catabolism
Increased acute phase protein synthesis by the liver
Interstitial fluid retention
Haemoconcentration
Serum electrolyte imbalance
Haemodynamic
Increased/decreased cardiac output
Hypotension
Tachycardia
Increased vascular permeability
Decreased vascular resistance
Immunological
Lymphokine production
Neutrophil leukocytosis
Transient depression of cell-mediated immunity (CMI)
Complement activation
Enhanced antibody production
Consumption of opsonins
Macrophage activation
Neutrophil activation and aggregation (adult respiratory distress syndrome – ARDS)

characterized by decreased cardiac output and hypotension, associated with severely impaired tissue perfusion, i.e., septic shock.

The haemodynamic responses are mediated by 'stress hormones' and by endogenous mediators. In fact, the haemodynamic changes associated with severe infections can be experimentally reproduced by the administration of endotoxin, tumour necrosis factor (TNF), C3a, and other mediators. Similarly, the hormonal and metabolic responses characteristic of the septic state can be provoked *in vivo* by administering TNF to experimental animals. Another aspect of the acute septic response is represented by the induced alterations affecting various immune defence mechanisms – cell-mediated and humoral immunity.

5.2 Cell-mediated immunity (CMI)

5.2.1 Lymphocyte counts and blastogenic responses

The modifications in the peripheral blood levels of total lymphocytes, helper T cells, suppressor T cells, and the proliferative response of peripheral blood lymphocytes *in vitro* to mitogenic stimuli (phytohaemagglutinin—PHA and concanavalin A—CON A), (see Chapter 9, Section 9.3.2) have been carefully studied in septic patients; serial determinations have been carried out immediately after the diagnosis of sepsis, and subsequently at weekly intervals. The number of total lymphocytes, T cells, and helper T cells have been shown to be significantly decreased in septic patients. The lymphocyte blastogenic response to PHA and to CON A during sepsis was also significantly depressed. Interestingly, in septic patients who survived the severe infections, the total lymphocyte count, the number of circulating helper T cells, and the suppressor T cells tended to return to normal values, whereas in non-survivors these cell counts remained persistently low. Prolonged depression of lymphocyte responses to PHA and CON A have been observed throughout the clinical course of severe infections, regardless of the clinical outcome; such depression has been shown to last for longer than four weeks. Recovery from a severe septic illness usually results in the normalization of the T cell profile in blood. We carried out prospective, sequential determinations of circulating total lymphocytes, T cells, and lymphocyte responses to PHA in surgical patients undergoing major operations, with a high risk of developing infections and septic complications. In patients undergoing resection of the colon and/or rectum, the occurrence of septic complications, within the first post-operative week (wound, urinary or respiratory tract infections or intra-abdominal sepsis) was associated with a prolonged depression of total lymphocyte counts and T cell counts. On the other hand, patients with an uncomplicated post-operative course showed the usual early post-operative (second to fourth post-operative day) and transient depression of CMI, promptly reversed after one to two weeks.

5.2.2 Skin tests

The depression of CMI in patients with sepsis is further documented by the observations of several authors regarding skin test responses (Nishijima *et al.* 1986). The presence of major infections at the time of admission to hospital or to the intensive care unit (ICU) is frequently accompanied by anergy to skin tests. Repeated skin testing in the ICU has shown that patients who were initially anergic remained immunologically unresponsive to the application/innoculation of antigens. Moreover, anergy to skin tests was associated with an increased mortality in septic patients. Prospective, serial skin testing of patients has suggested that severe infections can be responsible for cutaneous anergy. In fact, multiple factors are often responsible for the occurrence of cutaneous anergy, including advanced age, trauma, infection, malnutrition, and rarely, pre-existing immune depression.

5.3 Humoral immunity

5.3.1 Complement

In the presence of bacteria, 20 or more plasma proteins interact to coat the bacterial surface with antibody and C3b, one of the complement breakdown products. There are two pathways of complement activation. The first, called the *classical pathway* (see Chapter 1, p. 50), is initiated by interaction of a specific antibody with its corresponding antigen on the bacterial surface. This triggers an enzymatic cascade, beginning with the activation of C1 which in turn activates C4, C2, and C3. The major fragment of C3, C3b, can act, together with other factors, to amplify the cleavage of C3 and, therefore, to produce more C3b. The complement sequence can also be activated via the *alternative pathway*, which involves properdin, factor B, factor D, and C3, bypassing the early components of the classic pathway. Most bacteria initiate activation of C3 utilizing both pathways to a greater or lesser extent.

The coating of the bacterial surface by antibody (IgG) and C3b is called opsonization and is important because the deposited proteins serve as a means of recognition by phagocytic cells. The latter bind to the deposited complement and antibody by specific receptor sites which initiates the process of invagination and ingestion. Intracellular lysosomes fuse with the ingested phagosome to form a phagolysosome. The enzymes contained within the phagolysosome effect the destruction of the bacteria. The many humoral mediators and cellular inflammatory systems activated during sepsis are responsible for the development of septic shock. Immunological reactions causing complement activation occur early during sepsis and result in disturbances of haemodynamic flow and metabolic processes. Antibody-coated bacteria cause complement activation via the classical pathway. Experimental *in vivo* studies have shown that complement activation produces the typical systemic haemodynamic and visceral flow abnormalities seen in sepsis. In fact, in animal studies it has been possible to reproduce the characteristic haemodynamic changes of hyperdynamic sepsis, by causing progressive activation of complement; this results in redistribution of systemic blood flow and in a decrease of hepatic perfusion, similar to that which is observed during sepsis. Decreased visceral perfusion is well known to precede biochemical evidence of organ dysfunction; ischaemic organ injury associated with complement activation, and overt sepsis results in metabolic derangements. It has been postulated that organ injury in sepsis is predominantly due to a derangement of the micro-circulation. Complement-mediated activation of neutrophils results in margination, aggregation, and degranulation of these cells, with release of toxic oxygen metabolites and proteolytic enzymes. It has been shown in animal models of pulmonary injury that complement activation induces a sequence of events, resulting in damage to the capillary endothelium, deposition of fibrin and platelets, and a further amplification of the inflammatory response.

There is evidence that extensive complement activation generates substances which interfere with host defence mechanisms. Prolonged stimulation of neutrophils with the complement activation product C5a makes these cells less responsive to other chemotactic stimuli and may inactivate phagocytic cells, impairing their bactericidal capacity. It has been shown that other complement activation fragments may interfere with the anti-bacterial functions of neutrophils, causing increased susceptibility to infection in experimental animals by decreasing bacterial killing by neutrophils. Furthermore, C3d, another complement activation product, interferes with lymphocyte function.

It appears, therefore, that complement activation has opposing effects, namely, it can support non-specific defences against infections, but it may also contribute substances which are immunodepressive. Thus, the fine modulation of complement activation in sepsis by inhibitors of the complement system may be crucial in determining the net immunoregulatory effect of the complement system. The serum concentrations of some complement components are normal or raised during bacterial infections. If, however, infection progresses to the point of septic shock, the level of complement components become significantly reduced; C3, C4, and factor B are the most profoundly affected complement components (Fig. 5.1).

A significant correlation has been found between measured serum complement levels and the severity of infection. C3, C4, and factor B levels have been documented to be significantly reduced in patients with infections from Gram-negative organisms resulting in septic shock and a fatal outcome. On the other hand, patients with Gram-negative infections not resulting in septic shock or with nonfatal septic shock had normal or slightly low C3, C4, and factor B levels.

Whilst a definitive explanation for these immunological alterations is still lacking, the findings described above suggest an activation of the classical and/or alternative complement pathways by circulating immune-complexes and/or endotoxin. Certain products of complement activation (C3a and C5a) are known to be powerful anaphylotoxins having the ability to induce the release of a wide variety of vasoactive mediators from mast cells. Markedly elevated C3a levels have been found in patients with septic shock, and an inverse correlation between C3a levels and systemic vascular resistence was observed in these patients.

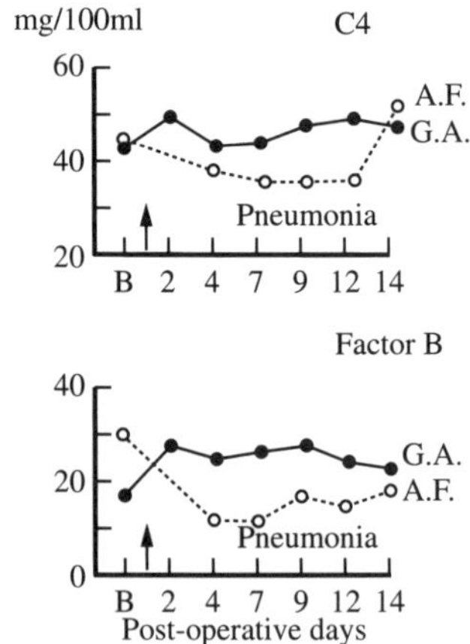

Fig. 5.1. Variations of C4 and factor B serum levels in two patients undergoing gastric resection for cancer. A.F., patient with post-operative pneumonia caused by *Klebsiella pneumoniae*; G.A., patient without any post-operative infections; B, baseline value; arrow, day of surgery.

5.3.2 Immunoglobulins

The plasma levels of immunoglobulins in patients with infections usually are within the normal range or above, as a result of enhanced stimulation of the humoral immune response. Some investigators have found that the serum levels of IgA, IgG, and IgM increased in patients who survived critical infections, whereas the immunoglobulins decreased progressively in patients who died from severe sepsis. Results of serial immunoglobulin determinations that we carried out in severely septic surgical patients confirm these observations. The antibodies, which are synthesized at an increased rate during infections, may be specific for the causative microorganism or they may be non-specific responses to the infectious disease (Nishijima *et al.* 1986).

5.3.3 Opsonins

Serum opsonins play a well-established role in host resistance against infections. Opsonins include serum factors which are either heat stable (immunoglobulins) or heat labile (complement), which have been demonstrated to adhere to pathogenic bacteria and to facilitate their phagocytosis and killing by neutrophils and monocytes. Consumption of antibodies and of complement during acute infection has been well documented and the ensuing defect of serum opsonizing capacity may partly explain the inability of the patients to control bacterial growth. Opsonization, ingestion, and killing by phagocytes are absolute requirements for resistence to extracellular bacteria. It has been reported that while opsonin serum levels usually rise following bacteraemia, as acute phase proteins, in some patients there is evidence of significant opsonin consumption. Consumption of opsonins, however, has been found to be associated with a high risk of bacteraemia only when neutrophil function was also abnormal. Based on these observations, therapeutic trials are currently under way, using the administration of high doses of polyvalent immunoglobulins, in an attempt to correct possible serum opsonic deficiency in septic surgical patients.

5.4 Macrophages

Macrophage activation occurs in surgically induced and traumatic wounds, as well as in infected tissues. Macrophage activation is initiated by a cascade of events starting with the activation of complement components by bacteria, by antigen-antibody complexes, and devitalized tissue. Released complement split products induce neutrophil chemotaxis, migration, and adhesion of leucocytes to the capillaries in the area of complement activation. Lymphokines are released by leucocytes, causing monocyte invasion and maturation into tissue macrophages. The complement split product C3b acts as an opsonin, binding both to the surface of bacteria and to the surface of the macrophage, facilitating phagocytosis and subsequent killing and digestion of bacteria. Oxygen-free radicals and lysosomal enzymes are released into the extracellular fluid during phagocytosis. The production of oxygen-free radicals, complement split products and lysosomal enzymes by macrophages may be extensive in major wounds and in infected tissues, leading to the release into the circulation of large amounts of molecules which may cause pulmonary endothelial damage, resulting in clinically overt respiratory insufficiency. Macrophages are an important source of TNF and IL-1, in response to endotoxin stimulation. These humoral mediators of sepsis released by macrophages are responsible for many of the homeostatic alterations observed during the septic syndrome. It has been shown that prevention of excessive macrophage activation is important for successful management of extensive tissue trauma and infection. This can be achieved by reducing macrophage-induced pulmonary damage and release of immunosuppressive products (Border 1988).

5.5 Neutrophils

Neutrophils play an important role in host defence against microbial invasion. They are activated during sepsis to produce maximal bactericidal activity. The manifestations of neutrophil activation include chemotaxis, aggregation, adherence, lysosomal degranulation, and superoxide radical

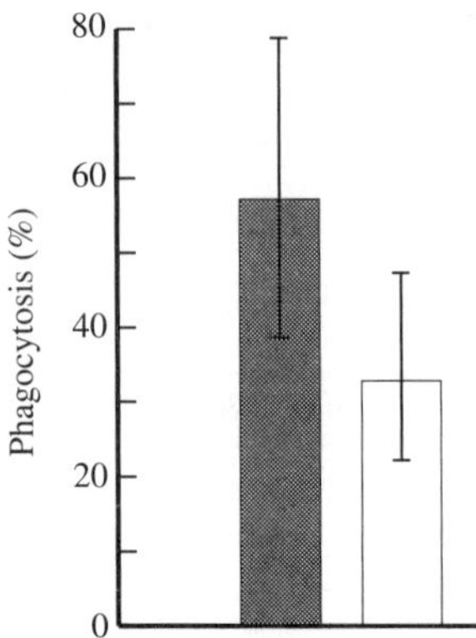

Fig. 5.2. Phagocytic activity of neutrophils in healthy subjects (shaded column) and in patients in septic shock (clear column). The difference is statistically significant.

production. Numerous endogenous mediators have been shown to induce activation of neutrophils during sepsis; these include TNF, endotoxin, C5a, and platelet-activating factor. Experimental studies have shown that in the early stage of infection, neutrophils are in a primed state, having the potential for enhanced oxidative activity, which can be used for bactericidal purposes, but which can also cause injury to the micro-circulation, particularly detrimental to the lung. Adult respiratory distress syndrome (ARDS) may be caused by the accumulation of neutrophils producing damage to the pulmonary micro-vasculature.

Neutrophil functions, however, may be impaired during infection. Neutrophil chemotaxis may decrease in patients who develop post-operative septic complications and it has been indicated that chemotaxis inhibiting factors are produced during the septic response. Neutrophils of patients with septic shock have an impairment of phagocytosis and microbial killing. A depression of bactericidal capability of neutrophils was shown to occur in patients who develop septic shock, preceding the onset of shock by several days (Fig. 5.2).

Neutrophils are primed in the early stage of infection and they are responsive to the complement split product C5a, which has been shown to aggregate neutrophils both *in vitro* and intravascularly *in vivo*. It has been suggested that neutrophil activation and aggregation during sepsis may cause micro-embolization, resulting in ischaemic tissue damage, which is characteristic of septic shock.

5.6 Humoral mediators and sepsis

Numerous studies carried out in recent years have indicated that the pathophysiological abnormalities observed during sepsis can be attributed to the multiple effects of humoral mediators released during infection. These mediators include endotoxin, complement activation fragments, tumour necrosis factor (TNF), the interleukins (ILs) and other activated mediators, the list of which is continuously being expanded. Multiple modifications of immunological, haemodynamic, hormonal, and metabolic homeostasis are induced by these mediators which are designed to ensure survival of the patient from infection.

The biological effects of endogenous mediators released during sepsis can be both beneficial and harmful. The beneficial effects consist in the elimination of the invading phatogens via the activation of immunological, cardiovascular, metabolic, and hormonal responses; the detrimental effects are represented by wasting of body lean tissue and by significant damage of target organs, such as the lung and the heart. (Michie *et al.* 1989)

5.6.1 Endotoxin

Endotoxin has been shown to exert multiple effects, in particular the activation of the complement cascade via the alternative pathway. Several other effects of endotoxin, including the induction of hyperpyrexia, protein catabolism, and refractory cardiovascular collapse, characteristic of septic shock, are mediated by other endogenous molecules which are produced by endotoxin-stimulated macrophages. In fact, endotoxin activates macrophages to release arachidonic acid metabolites—prostaglandins (PGE_2 and PGF_2), IL-1, and TNF.

5.6.2 Prostaglandins, IL-1 and TNF

Prostaglandins, among other activities, are currently believed to be the mediators of the febrile response at the central nervous system level.

IL-1 has very important properties relevant to host defences, including the stimulation of haemopoiesis, the activation of antibody production by B cells, induction of IL-2 and consequent stimulus to maturation of T and B lymphocytes. A number of the activities previously ascribed to IL-1, have recently been recognized to be due to TNF.

Currently, TNF is accepted as the principal molecule mediating the homeostatic alterations of sepsis (Michie *et al.* 1989). In fact, it has been observed that high doses of TNF administered to experimental animals induce haemodynamic collapse, metabolic alterations, and multiple organ failure (MOF). Systemic and visceral haemodynamic changes, which are typical of Gram-negative sepsis, can be observed following TNF injection.

TNF plasma levels are not generally elevated in patients presenting with the septic syndrome, because TNF has a very short half-life (a few hours), however, its biological effects are long lasting. Experiments with baboons, injected with *Escherichia coli*, indicate that high TNF levels are detectable in the plasma at the onset of septic shock. Nevertheless, the biological effects are prominent and prolonged, having significant effects long after its presence in the plasma is no longer demonstrable.

5.7 Septic shock

Septic shock can be defined as a generalized failure of tissue perfusion, resulting from infection, which manifests itself clinically by haemodynamic collapse and by metabolic evidence of impaired blood flow. The main clinical feature of septic shock is a reduction of arterial pressure, accompanied by increased anaerobic metabolism, which is usually documented by the presence of lactic acidosis. The haemodynamic and metabolic alterations characteristic of sepsis may present with different degrees of severity during the course of an infectious disease. There is a continuum of septic abnormalities from moderate infection to septic shock, the latter representing a late stage of septic alterations. Indeed, two phases of septic shock have been described: (1) *early septic shock*, featuring a hyperdynamic state (increased cardiac index, heart rate, oxygen consumption, fever, and tachypnoea); and (2) *late septic shock* featuring a hypodynamic state (decreased cardiac index, systemic vascular resistance, hypotension, and metabolic acidosis), which may proceed to irreversible cardio-circulatory collapse and death. Septic shock is a very severe complication of sepsis. It represents one of the most frequent causes of death in surgical patients, accounting for approximately 50 per cent of the causes of death in septic surgical patients being treated in intensive care units.

Several humoral mediators, which are activated during sepsis, are believed to cause septic shock. They include IL-1, TNF, and, especially, the complement split products C3a and C5a, whose serum levels are substantially elevated during septic shock.

5.8 Multiple organ failure (MOF)

About 10 years ago the clinical syndrome of MOF was described, indicating clinical and functional alterations associated with abnormalities of laboratory parameters which are representative of uncontrolled sepsis that has proceeded to cause failure of numerous organ systems. (Border 1988)

The organs/systems which are most commonly affected during sepsis are the lungs, the cardiovascular system, the kidneys, the liver, the digestive tract, and the coagulation system. The pathogenesis of MOF is attributed currently to the uncontrolled effect of septic mediators, such as TNF, the interleukins, activated complement, prostaglandins, oxygen-free radicals, and the coagulation system. MOF is also a very frequent cause of death in severely septic patients, accounting for approximately 50 per cent of the deaths.

Some important conclusions, from studies carried out during the last few years, concerning the relationships between infection and the septic response must be emphasized. Treatment of infection remains the cornerstone of the treatment of sepsis. However, the control of the infectious process does not always correct the problems of the altered septic response and of the ensuing MOF. It has become apparent that, in many severely ill septic patients, the main problem is control of the *septic state*, rather than the control of microbial infection *per se*. In fact, with the sensitive techniques available for the diagnosis of infection (radiological, bacteriological, and biochemical) and with the availability of effective antimicrobial therapy, the problem of infection is now much less important than that of sepsis. Clearly, progress in the treatment of septic patients will derive from the availability of more effective drugs and efficacious surgical techniques for treating infection, but especially from a better understanding of the pathophysiological mechanisms of uncontrolled sepsis.

5.9 Post-splenectomy infections

The risk of infection is significantly increased in patients after splenectomy. Estimates of the frequency of occurrence of post-splenectomy sepsis vary from 2.7 to 39 per cent, but almost all available controlled studies have found remarkably higher infection and mortality rates among younger patients. Post-splenectomy sepsis has been described as 'septicaemia, meningitis or pneumonia, usually fulminant, but not always fatal' (Singer 1973). More than 50 per cent of the cases of overwhelming sepsis occur within two years of splenectomy but it may also appear many years thereafter. Splenectomy in the paediatric patient seems to cause a rather selective type of immunodepression, characterized by increased susceptibility to infection by encapsulated organisms. It has been shown that over 50 per cent of cases of post-splenectomy sepsis involve pneumococcal organisms, followed in descending order of frequency by *Haemophilus influenzae*, *Neisseria meningitidis*, streptococci of the B-haemolytic group, *Escherichia coli*, and *Pseudomonas* species. Splenectomy causes a reduction in serum IgM and antibody levels, inhibits the specific IgM antibody response and abolishes the normal switching from the initial IgM response to the later IgG response. This results in poor opsonization and, therefore, reduced clearance of organisms as the liver can only remove well-opsonized bacteria from the blood.

The lack of a spleen-produced tetrapeptide, tuftsin, may be another factor in the initiation of post-splenectomy sepsis. This molecule promotes the phagocytic activity of polymorphonuclear leucocytes and disappears from the circulation six to eight weeks after splenectomy.

In view of the frequency and severity of post-splenectomy infections it is important to consider splenic salvage whenever possible, especially in children. The techniques which have been employed include non-surgical management, local pressure and topical haemostatic agents, splenorrhaphy, and 'cocooning' of the spleen in a polyglycolic acid mesh. When splenectomy is deemed necessary, prophylactic measures should be undertaken to avoid subsequent sepsis. All splenectomized patients should be given pneumococcal, meningococcoal, and *Haemophilus influenzae* vaccines. Patients undergoing elective splenectomy should receive the vaccines before surgery, and patients having emergency splenectomy for trauma should be vaccinated as soon as possible after surgery. All three vaccinations can be administered together, but they should not be given at the same time as chemotherapy or other immunosuppressive therapy. Prophylactic penicillin should be used in patients at high risk of infection, including children under five years of age and immunosuppressed patients. All patients should be instructed on the prompt recognition of and need for urgent treatment of infectious diseases.

Splenic autotransplantation has been advocated by some authors, although its efficacy in humans has not been proved. At least 30 g of splenic tissue should be transplanted into an omental pouch, the abdominal wall, or by intraperitoneal injection.

5.10 Immunotherapy of sepsis

5.10.1 Non-specific immunotherapy

New therapeutic strategies are being sought to modify the clinical course of severe sepsis. They have been developed in an attempt to improve defence mechanisms in septic patients, by stimulating the non-specific immune defences.

BCG and *Corynebacterium parvum* have been used to stimulate non-specific immune responses, with only modest results. Muramyldipeptide, another non-specific immunostimulatory drug, which is a mycobacterium cell wall component, has been shown to be effective if given in association with antibiotics. Gamma-interferon has been found to stimulate macrophages and monocytes *in vitro* and is currently being investigated in clinical studies and results are awaited with interest.

5.10.2 TNF blockade

A new therapeutic strategy, which is under study, consists of blocking TNF, which is recognized as the principal mediator of the septic state. Blockade of TNF has been experimentally obtained with anti-TNF antibodies and with glucocorticoids. However, neutralization of TNF requires that the blocking agents be administered at the beginning of infection, before the septic syndrome becomes clinically evident. These considerations may help explain why corticosteroids were reported to be effective in the cure of septic shock only rarely, and only when they were administered at the very beginning of the septic syndrome. The requirement of early administration of TNF-blocking agents renders such therapy not feasible in most clinical cases of septic shock. Alternative methods of blocking the systemic effects of TNF are currently being explored, based on the administration of drugs that inhibit the cyclo-oxygenase pathway.

5.10.3 Polyvalent immunoglobulins

Immunoglobulins (Ig) have been used for prophylaxis and for therapy of microbial infections. Experimental studies have shown that the intact Fc portion of IgG enhances opsonization and phagocytosis, and that therapy with IgG is effective in decreasing the mortality of septic animals. Human studies have been carried out in recent years to evaluate the effect of administering high doses of IgG intravenously for prophylaxis against

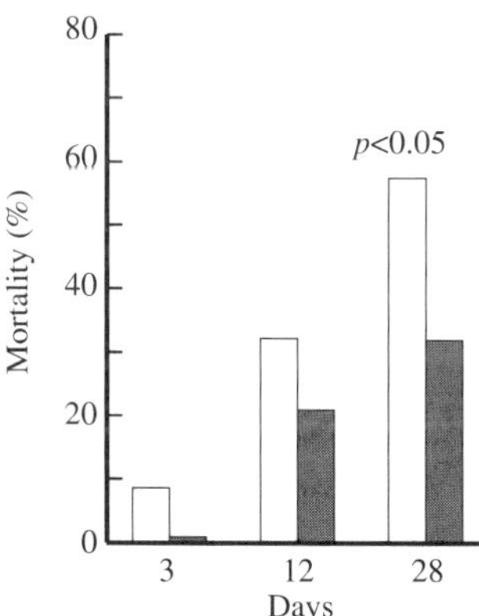

Fig. 5.3. Mortality of patients with severe surgical infections (sepsis score ≥ 20), undergoing intensive care treatment. Two groups of patients are reported: group 1, patients receiving conventional multi-modal treatment (clear columns); group 2, patients receiving the same treatment as those in group 1, but with high doses of intact IgG as additional therapy (shaded columns). Mortality of IgG-treated patients was significantly reduced after 28 days of treatment.

infections in high-risk trauma patients. Multiple trauma patients, receiving 36 g of polyvalent intact IgG prophylactically showed a decreased incidence of pneumonia as compared with patients receiving placebo. Recently, we carried out a prospective, randomized, placebo-controlled, double-blind study to evaluate the reduction in mortality with high doses of IgG with intact Fc portions given intravenously to severely septic surgical patients undergoing treatment in the intensive care unit. The results of our study showed that in surgical patients with very severe infections (initial sepsis score ≥20; Dominioni *et al.* 1987), treatment with high doses of IgG significantly reduced mortality from septic causes, especially reducing mortality in patients with septic shock (Fig. 5.3).

References and further reading

Border, J. R. (1988). Hypothesis: sepsis, multiple systems organ failure, and the macrophage. *Archives of Surgery*, **123**, 285–6.

Dionigi R. *et al.* (1987). Sepsis score and complement factor B for monitoring severely septic surgical patients and for predicting their survival. *European Surgical Research*, **17**, 269–80.

Dominioni L. *et al.* (1987). Sepsis score and acute-phase protein responses as predictors of outcome in septic surgical patients. *Archives of Surgery*, **122**, 141–6.

Michie H. R., Guillou P. S., and Wilmore D. W. (1989). Tumour necrosis factor and bacterial sepsis. *British Journal of Surgery*, **76**, 670–1.

Nishijima M. K. *et al.* (1986). Serial changes in cellular immunity of septic patients with multiple organ system failure. *Critical Care Medicine*, **14**, 87–91.

Singer D. B. (1975). Postsplenectomy sepsis. *Perspectives on Paediatric Pathology*, **1**, 285–91.

6
Nutrition and the immune response

O. Eremin and J. Broom

6.1 Protein energy malnutrition (PEM)

Protein energy malnutrition is a nutritional deficiency in which the protein and/or energy requirements are suboptimal. The clinical syndromes resulting from PEM vary according to the severity of the deficiency and the ratio of protein to energy in the diet. It has been recognized for many years that severe malnutrition predisposes to certain types of infection and that malnourished patients are often less able to cope with established infectious diseases than well-nourished individuals. This detrimental interaction between malnutrition and infection has been documented, particularly, in children living in underdeveloped countries. Similarly, there appears to be an increased incidence of sepsis occurring post-operatively in poorly nourished patients undergoing major surgery or recovering from severe trauma. In addition, patients with extensive malignant disease, who frequently show evidence of a defect(s) of host immunity, often have a variable degree of malnutrition. Such findings have led many observers to postulate that diet and nutritional status are closely interlinked with host resistance and defences, and that dietary factors possibly may modulate host defence mechanisms *in vivo*. Investigations in animals have shown that dietary alterations can influence significantly the immunological abnormalities seen in autoimmune diseases. Recent studies in humans indicate that calorie restriction can induce a variable clinical improvement in patients with rheumatoid arthritis. The precise interrelationships, however, between these various factors are not well characterized and further studies are needed to define more precisely the association between diet and immunity (see Chandra and Chandra 1986).

6.1.1 Cell-mediated immunity (CMI)

Alteration of lymphoid compartments

Severe PEM results in major alterations in morphology and microarchitecture of lymphoid tissues. The thymus is small, atrophied, and depleted of lymphocytes; the cortex is hypoplastic and poorly demarcated from the medulla. In rodents, severe PEM leads also to thymic epithelial involution, accumulation of lipid, and lack of cytoplasmic secretory vacuoles. Similarly, there is atrophy in other lymphoid organs—spleen, lymph nodes, tonsils, organ-associated lymphoid tissue—with particular depletion of thymus-dependent areas, e.g., peri-arteriolar cuff in spleen, paracortex in nodes, intraepithelial and lamina propria lymphocytes in gut-associated lymphoid tissue. Lymphopenia is not infrequent and the level of circulating mature T cells is reduced in the blood. This is partly a reflection of thymic atrophy and diminished thymic hormone secretion. Incubation of such blood lymphocytes *in vitro* with thymic hormones can increase, to a variable degree, the number of mature T cells. There is usually a reduction in the circulating levels of both T helper cells ($CD4^+$) and T suppressor/cytotoxic ($CD8^+$) lymphocyte subsets; the former being preferentially depleted. The residual (and depleted T lymphocytes) show deficits of homing to appropriate lymphoid target organs, e.g., lymph nodes. These alterations are outlined in Table 6.1.

Effect on functional properties

Apart from the obvious morphological changes described above, PEM is associated with significant alterations of CMI, documented by both *in vivo* and *in vitro* assays. *In vivo*, skin testing with both new (dinitrochlorobenzene) and recall antigens (streptokinase, streptodornase, candidin, mumps, etc.) reveals a variable response, with frequent cutaneous anergy, suggesting a defect of the delayed type hypersensitivity (DTH) response. The results obtained in animals, however, vary from species to species and are dependent on the acuteness and severity of protein deprivation. Despite this lack of specificity such observations provide an insight into the possible mechanisms underlying the anergy. Animal studies have documented a defective and diminished migration of mononuclear phagocytic cells to sites of inflammation. Not only is there a reduced number of antigen-presenting cells (APCs) but those that are present show low levels only of Ia antigen expression. *In vitro* testing, both in man and animals, reveals an impaired response to alloantigens (e.g., mixed lymphocyte culture (MLC)) and polyclonal activators (e.g., mitogens). Secretion of IL-1 by macrophages and IL-2 by T cells is diminished and the response of T helper cells to the cytokines is defective. Cell-mediated cytotoxic mechanisms (mediated by K, NK, T cells) are all substantially inhibited in PEM. The response of NK cells to interferon

Table 6.1. The Effect of PEM on immunity

Host defences studied	Effect documented
Humoral	
Blood B lymphocytes	N
Serum immunoglobulins	N/↑
Viral antibody titres	N/↓
Complement components	N/↓
Secretory IgA	↓
CMI	
Blood T lymphocytes ($CD3^+$, $CD4^+$, $CD8^+$)	↓
Lymphoid tissue T lymphocytes (thymus, spleen, nodes)	↓
Cytotoxic activities (K, NK, T)	↓
General reactivity (*in vitro*) (MLC, mitogens)	↓
General reactivity (*in vivo*) (DTH)	↓
Phagocytic activity (free radicals, enzymes)	↓
Cytokine production (IL-1, IL-2)	↓

N, normal; ↑, enhanced; ↓, reduced; K, killer cell; NK, natural killer cell; T, killer lymphocyte; MLC, mixed lymphocyte culture; DTH, delayed type hypersensitivity.

(IFN) is inhibited and the secretion of IFN-γ by activated T and NK cells is reduced. The phagocytic function of reticuloendothelial cells is usually normal but intracellular bactericidal activity, as determined by reduced free radical generation and decreased lysosomal enzyme production, may be abnormal, in particular in polymorphonuclear leucocytes (see Table 6.1). The spectrum and severity of abnormal immune reactivity in man is less well documented and characterized than the findings in experimental animals.

6.1.2 Humoral immunity

In contrast to the well-documented effects on CMI, abnormalities of humoral immunity are more variable and less well defined. The number of B lymphocytes in the circulation is within the normal range. The concentration of serum immunoglobulins is normal or elevated; the latter may be a reflection of recurrent infections that frequently accompany PEM.

Responses to specific antigens may be deficient in PEM, although a number of studies have failed to show a defective humoral response to vaccination in malnourished children. However, the titres of antibodies to viruses have been shown to be low in some malnourished infants and antibody production in response to thymus-dependent antigens is often defective. Animal studies reveal a defect of T helper ($CD4^+$) cells for IgG production and a reduced level of secretory IgA in the gut lumen in response to ingested antigens. Deficiencies in the production of secretory IgA in saliva, tears, and other secretions have been found in patients with PEM. Suppressive factors (inhibiting CMI) are found in the serum of some individuals with PEM. These factors, however, are poorly defined. Opsonic function of plasma from patients with PEM may be defective and complement components (C3, factor B, etc.) are usually low, presumably due to the increased production of immune complexes and their subsequent clearance from the circulation (see Table 6.1).

6.1.3 Autoimmunity

Prolonged PEM can modify substantially the onset, duration, and pathology of spontaneous rheumatoid disease in mice. PEM reduces the level of circulating immune complexes, production of autoantibodies, and deposition of complexes in various organs. CMI (as measured by *in vitro* responses to mitogens and alloantigens) returns to normal, and morphological abnormalities in lymphoid compartments (thymic atrophy, splenomegaly) are prevented or reduced. The few studies carried out in patients with autoimmune disease, manipulating dietary factors, have produced variable and inconclusive results.

6.2 Vitamins and immunity

Apart from hypovitaminosis A, isolated and/or gross deficiencies of vitamins in man are less frequent than previously, although they do occur in the under-developed world and possibly sub-clinically within our own hospital population. The prevalence of this latter situation is not known, not the least because of the inherent difficulty in assessing vitamin status for the vast majority of vitamins in man. Much of the published work on hypovitaminoses and the immune response is based on animal studies. Such studies are not readily extrapolated to man in that the functions of vitamins, in many aspects, are peculiar to the species concerned. In general, multiple vitamin deficiencies do not occur in man unless induced by iatrogenic means. In animals, severe depletion of vitamins has a pronounced inhibitory effect on various aspects of CMI and a less well-defined effect on humoral immune mechanisms (Table 6.2).

Table 6.2. The Effect of vitamin deficiency on immunity

Vitamin deficiency	**Host defences studied**	**Effect documented**
A, B	Humoral response (AB production)	↓
A, B, C	General reactivity (*in vitro*) (MLC, mitogens)	↓
A, B, C	General reactivity (*in vivo*) (DTH)	↓
A, C, D	Cytotoxic activities (NK, T, LAK)	↓
A, B, C	Phagocytic activity (free radicals, enzymes)	↓
D	Phagocytic activity (free radicals, enzymes)	↓
D	Cytokine secretion (IL-1, TNF)	↓
D	Cytokine secretion (IL-2, IFN-γ)	↑

↓, reduced; ↑, enhanced; AB, antibody; MLC, mixed lymphocyte culture; DTH, delayed type hypersensitivity; NK, natural killer cell; T, killer lymphocyte; LAK, lymphokine-activated killer cell;

NB Most of the above findings have been documented in animals.

6.2.1 Vitamin A

Vitamin A is involved in the control of cellular growth, and differentiation and gross deficiency of this vitamin has a prominent and widespread inhibitory effect on CMI. *In vitro* defects include reduced responses to mitogens and alloantigens, defective NK cell activity and T cell cytotoxicity, and impaired phagocytic activity by reticuloendothelial cells. *In vivo*, there are impaired responses to topical antigens similar to those seen in PEM. In animal models with autoimmune disease, Vitamin A deficiency enhances the process with the appearance of autoantibodies at an early stage and enhances the formation of immune complexes within the circulation. In terms of resistance to infection there is evidence that even mild hypovitaminosis A is detrimental. Increasing Vitamin A intake appears to have a beneficial effect on host defences by increasing NK cell activity, macrophage phagocytosis, and secretion of IL-1. It must be remembered, however, that this vitamin is particularly toxic when given in excess. The widespread effects of vitamin A deficiency are outlined in Table 6.2.

6.2.2 Vitamin B

Vitamin B6 and B12 deficiencies (folate deficiency mimics that of B12) are associated with abnormalities of CMI, similar to those seen with PEM. Vitamin B6, in particular, is essential for normal function of thymic epithelial cells; lack of B6 results in diminished secretion of thymic hormones. Low levels of B12 can inhibit the scavenging role of leucocytes, reduce the production of free radicals, and inhibit lytic enzyme secretion, thus resulting in defective bactericidal action. Deficiency of the B group of vitamins results in defective humoral responses with significantly reduced levels of antibody production (see Table 6.2).

6.2.3 Vitamin C

Isolated and severe vitamin C defects are rare but have been shown in humans to be associated with low levels of NK cell activity, and with inhibition of the inflammatory response. The primary effects of scurvy have been ascribed to impaired chemotactic activity of neutrophils and macrophages. Lack of vitamin C in animals can lead to defective activation of rodent spleen cells—assessed by *in vitro* responses of lymphocytes to mitogens and phagocytosis by macrophages. Vitamin C also has an important role, with other nutrients, in maintaining normal thymic function in rodents; scorbutic animals have lymphopenia and defective DTH responses. Deficiency of vitamin C was able to reduce the severity of autoimmune encephalomyelitis in mice. Vitamin C is essential only in man and the higher primates (and the guinea pig), and studies in other species must be interpreted with caution.

6.2.4 Vitamin D

Evidence is emerging that the vitamin D group, in particular calcitriol, can modulate substantially the immune system in man and animals (see Table 6.2). Receptors for vitamin D are widespread, being present on most cells, including lymphoreticular cells—monocytes-macrophages, activated circulating T and B lymphocytes, and mature T cells in the thymic medulla. Calcitriol, produced by the kidney (as well as by monocytes-macrophages), induces the production and release of cytokines (IL-1, TNF) by circulating blood monocytes and tissue macrophages. In addition, it also increases intracellular free radical release by these cells and in turn perturbates their cell membranes, increasing Fc receptor expression and enhancing the tendency for cell fusion. This results in significant activation of monocytes-macrophages, e.g., at sites of inflammation, resulting in enhanced phagocytosis and cytotoxicity. Calcitriol, on the other hand, inhibits the release of other cytokines (IFN-γ, IL-2) and decreases the further proliferation and function of activated NK, LAK, T cytotoxic cells, and CD4$^+$ T helper cells.

6.3 Trace element abnormalities

The role of trace elements (iron, zinc, copper, magnesium, and selenium) in maintaining the functional integrity of host defences is becoming more readily appreciated. Pure deficiencies, apart from iron, are rare; zinc and iron deficiency is not infrequently seen in patients with PEM, and selenium deficiency is usually seen in conjunction with lack of vitamin E. Prolonged intravenous hyperalimentation, with inappropriate dietary replacement, can lead to selective deficiencies of trace elements.

6.3.1 Iron

Iron deficiency

This is a common dietary problem, even in industrialized societies. Iron is essential for optimal activity of cells of the lymphoreticular system, regulating T cell membrane receptors/markers, T lymphocyte subsets and CMI responses (see Table 6.3). Iron deficiency may inhibit the scavenging activity of leucocytes by reducing the production and release of free radicals, thus reducing their ability to deal with infectious agents. The ability of iron-

Table 6.3. Effect of iron on immunity

Iron	**Host defences studied**	**Effect documented**
Deficiency	AB production	↓
	Phagocytic activities (free radicals)	↓
	General T lymphocyte reactivity (*in vitro*) (mitogens, MLC)	↓
	General T lymphocyte reactivity (*in vivo*) (DTH)	↓
	Lymphocyte cytotoxicities (NK, T)	↓
Excess	Phagocytic activities (free radical)	↓
	General T lymphocyte reactivity (in vitro) (mitogens, MLC)	↓
	Blood T lymphocyte $CD3^+$, $CD4^+$	↓
	$CD8^+$	↑
	Lymphocyte cytotoxicity (NK)	N

N, normal; ↓, reduced; ↑, enhanced; AB, antibody; MLC, mixed lymphocyte culture; DTH, delayed type hypersensitivity; NK, natural killer cell; T, T killer lymphocyte.

deficient individuals to mount an adequate humoral response to such agents, in particular viruses, has been shown to be defective with low titres of circulating anti-viral antibodies. Correspondingly, studies in man and animals have shown low levels of the free iron to be associated with a sub-optimal CMI: reduced cutaneous DTH responses to topical antigens, hyporeactivity of T lymphocytes to mitogens, defective NK, and T cytotoxic activity in animals. Repletion of iron stores results in reversal of this inhibition of host immunity. It is interesting to note, however, that with infection and activation of the immune system there is an immediate and substantial decrease in the circulating iron levels and in the capacity for iron binding and transport in the plasma. As in eukaryotes, prokaryotes have a dependency on maintaining a supply of iron for survival and a large number of their energy-dependent processes rely on iron metallo-enzymes. This reduction in circulating iron availability thus reduces the capacity for any invading organism to replicate whether dependent or independent of intact host defences.

Iron excess

Studies *in vitro* and *in vivo* (patients with B-thalassaemia, haemochromatosis) have confirmed the crucial interaction with, and modulation by excess iron on immune mechanisms (see Table 6.3). In general, phagocytosis and free radical release is defective in cells of the reticuloendothelial system. The $CD4^+$ lymphocyte subset is particularly sensitive to excess iron; substantial reduction in number and function of T helper cells have been documented in patients with iron overload. Correspondingly, there is an excess of circulatory $CD8^+$ lymphocytes. Ability of the lymphocytes to respond to mitogens and alloantigens is reduced (the latter appears to be related to HLA phenotype) but NK cell activity appears to be intact.

6.3.2 Zinc

This element is an essential metal for many cellular enzyme interactions involved in both anabolic and catabolic interactions, and in particular for nucleic acid transcription and replication. Inadequate tissue levels of zinc, therefore, have a profound biological effect, especially on lymphoid structure and function. Zinc deficiency produces a generalized atrophy of lymphoid tissue with a reduction in the thymic output of hormones and a resultant reduction in the number of mature T lymphocytes in the circulation. These changes are similar to those documented in mammals with PEM (see Table 6.1). These morphological and functional changes result in a significantly reduced CMI, both in man and animals, and are similar to the changes seen with PEM (see Section 6.1.1). Zinc therapy can ameliorate these abnormalities. Humoral immunity is affected to a variable degree. The number of B lymphocytes is usually unaffected, whilst antibody responses can be defective, particularly to T cell-dependent antigens. Severe depletion of zinc leads to defective leucocyte function – chemotaxis, Ia antigen expression and phagocytosis. Mild depletion, on the other hand, is beneficial whilst high levels of tissue zinc have been shown to inhibit leucocyte function in animals. Severe zinc deficiency is associated with an increased susceptibility to infections and defective healing of wounds. Rodents developing spontaneous autoimmune diseases, have the pathological process substantially modified if fed on a very low zinc diet, whilst still young, and before the development of the autoimmune disease process.

6.3.3 Copper

Copper deficiency is extremely rare in man except as the result of the administration of inappropriately constituted intravenous feeding regimens. It does, however, occur in animals. In such animals, copper deficiencies have been shown to modulate host defence mechanisms, e.g., mammals deficient in copper are more prone to certain types of bacterial infections. Data from experimental studies, however, reveal variable results, with an inhibition of both CMI and humoral immunity as well as defective leucocyte function – reduced Ia antigen expression, inhibition of phagocytosis, and defective lytic enzyme production. Again, the requirement for copper is in relation to metallo-enzyme systems in the energy transduction processes and deficiencies will tend to mimic the effects seen with PEM (see Table 6.1).

6.3.4 Magnesium

Although magnesium deficiency has been documented in both man and animals, its effect on host defences has been studied only in the latter. Magnesium is essential for many biological processes, including growth, differentiation, and activation of cells of the lymphoreticular system. Severe lack of magnesium affects both antibody production and cell-mediated functions. Because of its involvement as an active compound in many intracellular reactions, its deficiency tends to produce disturbances of the immune system, comparable to that outlined for the other metals above.

6.3.5 Selenium

This is an essential component of the enzyme glutathione peroxidase and like vitamin E, is an anti-oxidant and protects against lipid peroxidation of cell membranes. Both selenium and vitamin E act as scavengers of free radicals and thus prevent oxidation of membrane polyunsaturated fatty acids (PUFA). Animal studies show that deficiencies of selenium (often with vitamin E) result in abnormalities of reticuloendothelial cell function e.g. defective phagocytosis and free radicle production. There is some evidence to suggest that it may have a role in maintaining a normal thymic epithelium.

6.4 Lipids and immunity

In Western societies high cholesterol/high fat diets are believed to be responsible for, or predispose to, the development of a number of disease processes—atherosclerosis and its attendant cardiovascular morbidity, diabetes, and possibly cancer. In the latter, modulation of host immunity may be an important underlying mechanism in the development of the malignant process, e.g., in breast, colo-rectal and prostatic carcinoma, both in man and experimental animals. In recent years, data has accumulated from human and animal studies showing that lipids can modulate the immune response. (Johnston 1986) The effect, however, depends on the type of fat ingested, the duration of feeding, and the particular lymphoreticular compartment investigated. Even the amount of body fat present has been suggested to have a role in modulating the immune system, in that genetically obese mice have been found to have some alteration of immunity e.g. reduced DTH responses and prolongation of skin graft survival.

6.4.1 Deficiency of lipids

Cholesterol, high density lipoproteins, and fatty acids are essential for normal function of the immune system. Studies in rodents reveal that feeding animals a diet deficient in essential fatty acids (EFA) can result in alterations of the immune system. Lymphoid atrophy has been documented, as well as reduced DTH responses, and a defective humoral response to antigens. In the latter, the responses elicited can vary, depending on the route of entry of the antigen. Essential fatty acid deficiencies have been reported in patients receiving both parenteral and naso-enteric support with inadequately designed diets. EFAs themselves are important precursors for the synthesis of intracellular and extracellular messengers and signals—prostaglandins and leucotrienes. Deficiencies in the precursors of these signal molecules have effects on leucocyte function through the absence of substrate for phospholipase A2 activity which is a key enzyme for signal cell transduction in both leucocyte and monocyte activation. As part of the acute inflammatory response is dependent on the production of the prostaglandin series, reduction in the precursor supply will have a beneficial effect on autoimmune disease. In rodent models with autoimmune disease, a low fat diet delays the onset of the disease process, improves survival; histologically there is a diminution in the infiltration of affected organs by lymphocytes.

6.4.2 Excess of lipids

Excess cholesterol, high density lipoproteins (HDLs), very low density lipoproteins (VLDLs), and PUFAs, either in *in vitro* assay systems or *in vivo* in animal models, can modulate substantially various aspects of the immune response—CMI and reticuloendothelial function. In addition, the levels of VLDL and HDL also will affect the system indirectly by modulating the transport of cholesterol to and from peripheral sites of cholesterol metabolism. Cholesterol and PUFA are believed to affect host defences by: (1) Altering the lipid content and fluidity of cell membranes, thereby affecting cell surface receptors, membrane metabolism during cell contact and activation. Activated lymphocytes show a marked turnover in membrane fatty acids with an increased incorporation of PUFA in this state; (2) Acting as molecular mediators; arachidonic acid which arises from essential fatty acids (e.g., linoleic) is an important precursor of the prostaglandins and related eicosanoids (e.g., leucotrienes). The prostaglandins are known to have significant inhibitory effects on host defences. Stimulation of lymphoreticular cells by antigens or mitogens induces the production and release of prostaglandins. The released prostaglandins inhibit, directly or via activation of suppressor lymphocytes, T and B lymphocyte reactivity and the release of various lymphokines. Prolonged exposure to excess PUFA, as well as saturated fatty acids, induce lymphoid atrophy in experimental animals and inhibit substantially CMI. The latter effects are documented both *in vitro*: reducing responses of lymphocytes to mitogens and alloantigens; and *in vivo*: reducing cutaneous DTH responses to topical antigens, prolongation of allogeneic grafts, inhibition of graft versus host disease, and ameliorating the severity of certain autoimmune diseases. High fat (PUFA, saturated) diets enhance the autoimmune processes, e.g., increase the level of circulating immune complexes and their depositions in various organs, and decrease survival. Preliminary studies in man have shown that fish oil diets can improve clinically some patients with rheumatoid arthritis. This whole area of PUFA and saturated fat intake, in relation to immune function, however, is currently being actively debated. Their exact roles, in either stimulating or inhibiting aspects of the immune response, presently is under active investigation.

6.5 Summary

The current state of knowledge of the various nutrients (proteins, fats, minerals, and vitamins) on host defences in man is fragmentary, inadequately documented, and open to conflicting interpretations. The investigations into the relationship between nutrition and immunological function have been neither systematic nor comprehensive, and in many instances carried out in various animal models. None of the major nutrients nor trace elements have been studied to any great depth and in isolation from the effects of other nutrients. However, in spite of the reservations expressed above, the studies which have been performed to date do suggest that various elements of the diet, singly or in combination, appear to have substantial effects on both cell-mediated and humoral immunity. A great deal of work needs to be done to clarify the suggested relationships outlined above, but offers the exciting prospect of possible modulation of host defences, through dietary intervention, both as a preventative measure and as innovative therapy in the major diseases affecting man.

References and Further reading

S. Chandra and R.K. Chandra (1986). Nutrition, immune response and outcome. *Progress in Food Nutrition Science*, **10**, 1–65.

D. Hwang (1989). Essential fatty acids and immune response. *The FASEB Journal*, **3**, 2052–61.

P.V. Johnston (1986). Dietary fat, eicosanoids and immunity. *Advances in Lipid Research*, **21**, 103–41.

7
Therapy and the immune response

O. Eremin

7.1 Introduction

As surgeons and clinicians, we employ various forms of therapy which, although regarded as essential for the patient's well-being, may in themselves have a detrimental effect on host defences. Some of the morbidity (e.g., sepsis) seen in the post-operative period after major surgery may, in part, be due to inhibition of the immune response in the peri-operative period, as a result of the anaesthesia given and the nature of the surgery carried out. Recently, a number of retrospective studies have suggested that blood transfusions may be immuno-inhibitory and detrimental to the survival of patients undergoing surgery for malignant disease. In patients with cancer, increased numbers of malignant cells enter the circulation during anaesthesia and surgery; inhibition of anti-tumour host defences during this phase may result in the enhanced metastatic dissemination of malignant cells and the establishment of occult tumour deposits. Studies in animals tend to substantiate such a hypothesis. Many of the drugs (e.g., chemotherapeutic agents) used to treat cancer and external beam radiotherapy, have well-documented and prolonged detrimental effects on aspects of the immune response. Recently, biological immune modulators (interferons, interleukins) have been introduced into clinical practice. Recombinant technology is producing an ever increasing variety of substances in vast quantities for potential use against cancer. The trainee surgeon must be familiar with the 'tools of his trade' and be aware of these exciting new developments in biology. This chapter will discuss in general terms, the modulation of the immune response

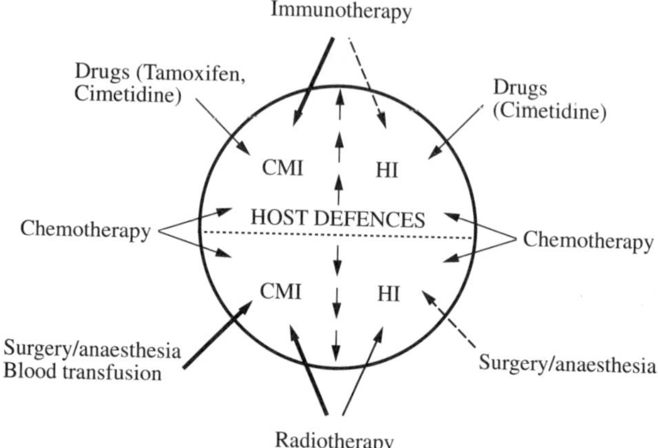

Fig. 7.1. Modulatory effects of various forms of therapy on host defences. ➞, marked effect; →, moderate effect; - - -➞ possible effect; CMI, cell-mediated immunity; HI, humoral immunity.

by various forms of therapy (Fig. 7.1). Thermal damage and more protracted forms of injury are discussed in Chapter 4, the effects of corticosteroids and immunosuppressive drugs are dealt with in Chapters 1 and 2. A detailed account of cytokines is found in Chapter 1.

7.2 Anaesthesia and surgery

Substantial evidence has accumulated showing that anaesthesia and surgery, both in man and experimental animals, can modulate (usually inhibit) the immune response. Anaesthesia and surgery induce a complex neuroendocrine-metabolic response, which has been postulated to play a major role in this modulation of host defences (Stevenson *et al.* 1990).

7.2.1 Anaesthesia

Almost one hundred years ago, it was documented that ether was able to induce a leucocytosis shortly after initiation of anaesthesia and that (with the added effect of surgery) this leucocytosis could persist for several days. Several more recent studies have confirmed this neutrophil leucocytosis following anaesthesia; others, however, have failed to document this increased circulating white cell count with anaesthesia alone. Some anaesthetic agents (e.g., Halothane) have been shown to produce a lymphopenia, albeit transient. *In vitro* studies have shown that nitrous oxide and thiopentone can inhibit neutrophil chemotaxis. Although Halothane has been found not to have the latter effect *in vitro*, paradoxically, *in vivo* (skin windows) studies have documented an inhibition of neutrophil migration to sites of inflammation.

Inhibition of *cell-mediated immunity (CMI)*, as assessed by *in vitro* reactivity to mitogens and alloantigens in both man and experimental animals, is well documented. Inhibition of reactivity can be detected several hours after induction of anaesthesia and may persist for up to two weeks post-anaesthesia. Few studies have evaluated cytotoxic mechanisms but suppression of T cytolytic and NK activity *in vitro* have been reported. The mechanism for this depression of CMI is unclear, but *in vitro* studies have shown that some of the commonly used agents (Halothane, nitrous oxide, diethyl ether, etc.) are anti-mitotic to a variety of cells in culture and inhibit both RNA and protein synthesis of mitogen-stimulated human blood lymphocytes.

The effect of anaesthetic agents on *humoral immunity* is less well studied but appears to be less readily immuno-inhibitory. Diminished levels of complement components (C3 and C5) have been described with Halothane anaesthesia. Some studies in animals have noted reduced production of antibodies for 48 hours post-anaesthesia. Other workers, on the other hand, have failed to detect any effect on humoral immunity with either ether or Halothane.

7.2.2 Surgery

Although anaesthesia does have an effect on the immune response, it is less well documented, less consistent, and much less severe than that associated with major surgery. The more extensive the surgery the more pronounced the modulation of host defences. The pain and emotional arousal associated with anaesthesia and surgery, as well as the stimuli emanating from volume, temperature, and chemoreceptors, alterations of circulating levels of glucose and amino acids, etc., induces a complex neuroendocrine-metabolic response. The latter results in the release of many hormones—catecholamines, cortisol/ACTH, endogenous opiates, vasopressin, etc. The tissue damage experienced in major surgery, as well as other factors (hypoxia, the enhanced hormone output, etc.), results in the increased production of cytokines (e.g. IL-1), biological enhancers of inflammation (leucotrienes) and the prostaglandins. IL-1, released at the site of injury and by monocytes-macrophages is a powerful stimulus (as is IL-6) in enhancing hepatic release of acute phase reactants, e.g., C reactive protein, factor B and other complement components, which are important in antibody-antigen interactions and clearance of immune complexes by the reticulo-endothelial system, inhibition of proteolytic enzymes, as well as being important chemo-attractants for leucocytes. IL-1 is an important growth factor for T helper cells and subsequent secretion of IL-2 and natural killer

(NK) cell activity. The prostaglandins and corticosteroids, on the other hand, are powerful inhibitors of the immune response.

Cell mediated immunity (CMI)

Although some studies have failed to elicit any alteration in the number of circulating lymphocytes, the majority of investigations have documented a lymphopenia, particularly following major surgery. In these latter studies, substantial reductions have been recorded in mature T lymphocytes ($CD3^+$) and T helper ($CD4^+$) subsets, occurring within 24 hours of surgery and persisting for up to one week following surgical trauma. There has not always been a corresponding alteration of the $CD8^+$ subset, but both a reduction and elevation have been detected. Inhibition of lymphocyte responses *in vitro* to polyclonal activators and alloantigens has been documented in numerous studies (man and animals). The inhibition has been recorded as early as two hours following commencement of surgery and has persisted for several days post-surgery; in some cases the hyporeactivity has lasted for up to two weeks. Concomitantly, these anergic lymphocytes show a marked reduction of lymphokine secretion (IL-2, IFN-γ). Inhibition of cutaneous delayed type hypersensitivity (DTH) responses to topical antigens has been monitored both in man and experimental animals. The few studies done to date on T cell cytotoxicity have revealed a defective killer cell activity. A number of studies have evaluated NK cell activity, revealing an inhibition of natural cytotoxicity, detected 24 hours post-trauma and persisting for one to two weeks following surgery (see Table 7.1).

Table 7.1. Effect of surgery on cell-mediated immunity*

Where Assessed	How assessed	Effect documented
In vivo	White cell count	↑
	T lymphocytes ($CD3^+$, $CD4^+$)	↓
	T lymphocytes ($CD8^+$)	↑/↓
	Macrophage-suppressor cell	↑
	DTH	↓
	Cytokines (IL-1, IL-6)	↑
In vitro	Mitogen, MLC	↓
	Killer cells (T, NK)	↓
	Macrophage phagocytosis	↑/↓
	White cell chemotaxis	↓

* Effect can be detected two hours post-surgery (e.g., mitogens) and last for up to two weeks (e.g., NK).

↑, enhanced; ↓, decreased; DTH, delayed type hypersensitivity; MLC, mixed lymphocyte culture; NK, natural killer cell; T, specific T killer cell.

Humoral immunity

Most investigations have failed to detect any alteration in the number of circulating B lymphocytes following surgery; a few, however, have recorded a reduction of B lymphocytes. Whilst circulating levels of immunoglobulin, e.g., IgG, have been shown to fall intra-operatively, significant changes in plasma concentrations have not been consistently documented post-operatively. Similarly, the ability to generate an antibody response to, for example, sheep red blood cells has produced variable results, depending on the animal model employed—enhanced responses in mice and rats, no alteration with chickens, and a fall in the guinea pig.

Reticuloendothelial system

Leucocytosis (neutrophilia) is a well-documented occurrence post-operatively and is probably due to the action of increased IL-1 secretion in association with tissue injury. There is some evidence to suggest, however, that both the neutrophil and monocyte show altered functional activity following surgery. Although enhanced phagocytosis in the immediate post-operative period has been detected, as has secretion of lysozyme, inhibition of reticuloendothelial cell function is not an infrequent finding—defective mobilization *in vivo* and deficient clearance of circulating aggregates, inhibition of chemotaxis, and phagocytosis *in vitro* (see Table 7.1).

The precise immunological mechanisms responsible for the alterations described above are not well understood, but *suppressor factors* (cellular and/or humoral) are believed to play a key role. A variety of serum inhibitory factors have been detected in patients and animals subjected to surgery. Some of these are normal constituents with a substantially increased output induced by surgery (adrenocorticoid hormones, α-2-macroglobulin, C reactive proteins), others appear to be new molecules (high molecular weight lipoproteins, low molecular weight globulin). The temporal distribution of these substances, however, does not closely correlate with the presence of immune suppression. Both suppressor T lymphocytes and monocytes-macrophages have been implicated in the suppression of the immune response after anaesthesia and surgery. Convincing evidence has been obtained, both in man and animals, that many of the inhibitory processes described above are mediated by monocytes-macrophages.

Monocytes-macrophages have been shown to inhibit killer cell activity (T, NK), responses to alloantigens and to inhibit the release of IL-1 (macrophages) and IL-2 (T helper cells), and to secrete substantial amounts of prostaglandins, e.g., PGE_2. The prostaglandins have been shown to inhibit/modify various immune processes—inhibit the release of IL-1 by and the surface expression of Ia antigens on monocytes-macrophages, activate $CD8^+$ lymphocytes, and suppress the release of IL-2 by $CD4^+$

lymphocytes. Probably, more than one suppressor mechanism is in operation during and following surgery.

7.3 Radiotherapy and chemotherapy

7.3.1 Radiotherapy

Over the past two decades a number of studies have documented the substantial and prolonged lymphopenia which results following radiotherapy. The circulating lymphocyte count may be reduced by up to 75 per cent shortly after completion of therapy. Both T and B lymphocyte subsets appear to be very radio-sensitive. However, the fall in circulating T lymphocytes is usually more profound and the effect more chronic. Diminished T cell counts have been recorded in patients up to one to two years post-radiotherapy, but B cell counts tend to return to pre-treatment values much sooner, usually within six months. Human T lymphocyte subsets show a differential sensitivity. The more 'mature' T lymphocytes (expressing high affinity receptors for sheep erythrocytes) are relatively radio-resistant. Both T helper and T suppressor lymphocytes have been shown to be sensitive; some studies have suggested that the T suppressor cell population is more radio-sensitive. NK and K cells are reduced in the circulation following radiotherapy but their recovery is usually relatively rapid and numbers return to pre-treatment levels after several months. There have been few functional studies carried out. In general, the lymphopenia is associated with a lymphocyte hyporeactivity, as measured by *in vitro* responses to mitogens. Studies in rodents have shown that high doses of radiation (400 cGy) reduces substantially, and for several weeks, the ability of spleen mononuclear cells to secrete IL-2. Low doses (100 cGy), on the other hand, have been shown to enhance the secretion of IL-2. Several studies have shown that the critical factor inducing lymphopenia appears to be the volume of blood irradiated. Comparable findings have been documented with irradiation of the pelvic organs and the chest area. Irradiation of the thymus does not appear to be more detrimental in terms of the lymphopenia detected.

7.3.2 Chemotherapy

It has become well recognized that anti-cancer drugs may have profound effects on the immune response. Chemotherapeutic drugs have been shown to both inhibit and augment host defences, depending on the regimen employed (dose and mode of drug delivery), type of antigen and its route of administration, and the immune parameters studied. Studies in tumour-bearing rodents, given cyclophosphamide, vinca alkaloids or adriamycin have demonstrated an enhanced and accelerated tumour regression but only in animals with intact immune mechanisms, suggesting an augmentation of anti-tumour defences, e.g., enhanced production of cytotoxic T cells, abrogation of suppressor mechanisms. Minor differences in the structure of the drugs given can have profound effects on the immune responses elicited; selective effects on CMI and humoral immunity by vincristine and vinblastine respectively, specific action on T cell subsets by the hepatic metabolite of cyclophosphamide (4-hydroperoxy-cyclophosphamide) and lack of action by the parent drug itself.

Inhibition

Both *humoral* and *cellular immune* functions are inhibited to a variable degree by a variety of chemotherapeutic agents (see Table 7.2). A reduced ability by B lymphocytes, albeit temporary, to mount an appropriate antibody response to antigens, particularly if both the chemotherapeutic drugs and antigen are given at the same time, has been documented with adriamycin, cyclophosphamide, *cis*-platinum, and vinblastine. Chemotherapeutic drugs not only reduce circulating levels of leucocytes (by affecting stem cell maturation in the bone marrow) but also induce functional disturbances, e.g., impaired phagocytic capability and release of lytic enzymes. Chemotherapeutic drugs which inhibit DNA synthesis have been shown to reduce monocyte migration to sites of inflammation. *Suppression of CMI* has been documented *in vivo* (cutaneous anergy with topical antigens— cyclophosphamide), and *in vitro* (hyporeactivity of lymphocytes to polyclonal mitogens and alloantigens—cyclophosphamide, *cis*-platinum, 5-fluorouracil-(5-FU)). Inhibition of NK and K cell activities have been demonstrated with a number of chemotherapeutic agents, e.g., adriamycin, cyclophosphamide, vincristine, methotrexate, and mitomycin C. Other cytotoxic mechanisms have not been well studied (see Table 7.2).

Augmentation

A large number of studies, both in man and animals have documented augmentation of immune responses with chemotherapy (see Table 7.2). *Enhanced antibody production in vivo* has been found with cyclophosphamide, melphalan, and *cis*-platinum. There is some evidence that *cis*-platinum may enhance the antigenicity of membrane antigens, in particular tumour associated antigens. A wide range of chemotherapeutic drugs (adriamycin, cyclophosphamide, methotrexate, mitomycin C, *cis*-platinum, vincristine, and 5-FU) have been shown to *augment various aspects of CMI*—cutaneous DTH responses, increased T cell cytotoxicity. The latter is believed to be an important factor in the enhanced anti-tumour responses (with associated regression of tumours) demonstrated in animal tumour models given either cyclophosphamide, vinblastine or adriamycin. These drugs have been shown to have selective effects on CMI. Studies in animals have demonstrated that activation of macrophage precursors as well as removal/inhibition

Table 7.2. Effect of chemotherapeutic drugs on host defences

	Host defences		
Chemotherapeutic drug	**CMI**		**Humoral immunity**
Cyclophosphamide	DTH	↑/↓	AB production ↑/↓
	Macrophage phagocytosis	↓	
	NK/K cytotoxicity	↓	
	Lymphocyte reactivity (mitogens, MLC)	↓	
	T cytotoxicity	↑	
	Suppressor cells (T)	↓	
Adriamycin	NK/K cytotoxicity	↓	AB production ↓
	T cytotoxicity	↑	
	Macrophage cytotoxicity	↑	
	Suppressor cells (T)	↓	
	Cytokines (IL-1, IL-2)	↑	
CIS-Platinum	DTH	↑	AB production ↑/↓
	T cytotoxicity	↑	
	Macrophage phagocytosis	↓	
	Lymphocyte reactivity (mitogens, MLC)	↓	
Vincristine Vinblastine	DTH	↑	AB production ↓
	NK/K cytotoxicity	↓	
	T cytotoxicity	↑	
5-FU	Lymphocyte reactivity (mitogens, MLC)	↓	
	DTH	↑	N.E.
	T cytotoxicity	↑	
	NK/K/LAK cytotoxicity	↑	
Mitomycin C Methotrexate	DTH	↑	
	T cytotoxicity	↑	N.E.
	NK/K cytotoxicity	↓	
Melphalan	Cytokine (IL-2)	↑	AB production ↑

↑, enhanced; ↓, reduced; N.E.: Not established; NK/K, natural killer/killer cells; T, T killer lymphocyte; LAK, lymphokine-activated killer cell; DTH, delayed type hypersensitivity; AB, antibody; MLC, mixed lymphocyte culture.

of regulatory T cells, as a result of adriamycin therapy, results in the pronounced and widespread enhancement of T cell cytotoxicity. On the other hand, cyclophosphamide exerts its augmenting effect, via its hepatic metabolite, by inhibiting the maturation/proliferation of precursors and inducers of T suppressor cells. Monocyte-macrophage numbers, as well as cytotoxicity, are enhanced by adriamycin. The latter also induces the release and secretion of cytokines – IL-1 by macrophages and IL-2 by T helper cells, and prostaglandins – PGE_2. Treatment of mice with low doses of other drugs (e.g. melphalan, cyclophosphamide) also enhances the secretion of IL-2 by spleen cells. Augmentation of NK cell activity has been described in some animal models. Recent studies in man suggest that treatment with 5-FU over several weeks may result in the augmentation of LAK cell activity (see Table 7.2). Further careful studies are necessary to define more precisely the possible immunomodulatory role of various chemotherapeutic combinations used in cancer treatment.

7.4 Blood transfusion

It is now generally accepted that some patients given blood transfusions prior to receiving renal allografts may have a prolongation of graft survival, in the presence of concomitant drug-induced immunosuppression. The transfusions must be given before (several weeks) or during surgery to obtain this beneficial effect. Various mechanisms have been postulated to explain this enhanced allograft survival, including the induction of tolerance to the grafted alloantigens and the generation of anti-idiotype antibodies. The transfusion of allogeneic blood cells, particularly the buffy coat containing leucocytes, has been shown to have a varied and complex inhibitory effect on the recipient's host defences. A reduction of general lymphocyte reactivity (detected *in vitro* by mixed lymphocyte culture (MLC) and mitogen assays) has been documented in a number of studies, as well as substantial reductions of NK cell activity. *Suppressor mechanisms* (cellular and humoral) are activated and are postulated to inhibit cell-mediated immunity. Both T lymphocytes and monocytes-macrophages have been invoked as the suppressor cells, mediating suppression through the release of various factors, e.g., α-2-macroglobulin, prostaglandins, etc. Animal studies suggest that blood transfusions induce both non-specific and antigen-specific suppression of immune reactivity.

Over the past decade, a number of publications, based on retrospective analyses, have reported that patients undergoing curative surgery for malignant disease and receiving peri-operative blood transfusions, have a reduced disease-free interval and survival. This has been documented in patients with various types of solid cancers – colon-rectum, breast, lung, and soft tissue sarcomas. A smaller, but still substantial number of analyses, on the other hand, have failed to find statistically convincing data in patients with similar pathological types of tumours.

Studies in rodents, however, have produced convincing evidence that blood transfusions, in particular the use of allogeneic white blood cells and/or plasma, prior to or just shortly after innoculations/transplantations of tumour cells, results in an enhanced growth and metastatic dissemination. Care must be taken in extrapolating data from animal studies to man. Also, other factors in man, e.g., skill of the surgeon, general well-being of the patient, extent of local growth, etc., make the interpretation of the results difficult and the analysis complex. Properly established and performed prospective trials, which are currently being established, should eventually provide the necessary answers. It is hoped that such studies will delineate more precisely the role, if any, of red blood cells, leucocytes, and plasma in altering disease-free interval and survival in patients undergoing curative surgery for malignant disease. For a more detailed description of the effects of blood transfusion on the surgical patient see Collins (1989).

7.5 Immunotherapy

7.5.1 Cytokines

Interferons (IFNs)

In the past decade IFNs, initially produced from banked white blood cells or lymphoblastoid cell lines, and more recently by recombinant DNA technology (RIFN), have been used to treat a variety of both solid cancers and lympho-haematological malignancies. IFNs, have a widespread and pronounced effect on cells of the lymphoreticular system—enhancement of NK, LAK and cytolytic T cell activities, stimulation of monocytes-macrophages (Fc IgG receptor expression, phagocytosis, cytotoxicity), regulation of Ig secretion by B lymphocytes, and increased cell surface expression of class I and II antigens. An important mechanism of this modulating effect is due to the release of and/or potentiation of the action of various other cytokines, e.g., IL-1, IL-2, TNF, and CSF (see Chapter 1 for further details). Natural and RIFN subtypes have been used predominantly in clinical trials, although immune or IFN-γ (released by activated T and NK cells) has the widest and most pronounced immunomodulatory effects. The IFNs, through their action as down-regulators of cellular genes, have induced stasis and/or regression in some animal tumours. Studies in man have shown the most benefit in patients with haematological malignancies—Hairy cell leukaemia; chronic myeloid leukaemia and myeloma, and Kaposi's sarcoma. The response of the common solid cancers has been disappointing, both with RIFN-α and RIFN-γ. Side-effects, resembling a flu-like illness are common (possibly due to a concomitant release of IL-1), and a wide spectrum of toxicity has been documented. The effects on host defences are variable, often contradictory and dependent on the dose and mode of IFN administration. Both inhibition and enhancement of NK cell activity have been documented. The latter effect has not usually persisted with prolonged therapy. Combination therapy with chemotherapeutic drugs and other cytokines (IL-2, TNF) are currently in progress. The rationale for such combinations is based on the immunomodulatory effects described above.

Interleukin-2 (IL-2)

IL-2 is a 15 500 Da glycoprotein produced by activated T lymphocytes (alloantigen-mitogen stimulated) and NK cells. It interacts with receptors for IL-2 on surface membranes and induces transmembrane signals through the B chain of the high affinity receptor. It enhances the proliferation and activity of a variety of T cell subsets (helper, cytotoxic cells), NK and LAK cells. The latter are believed to be derived from precursors of NK cells, but the precise cell lineage is uncertain. Recently, IL-2 has been documented to interact with B cells and monocytes-macrophages. IL-2 induces the secretion of IFN-γ, TNF, and IL-1, and is itself modulated by these lymphokines. During the past decade Rosenberg and his colleagues in the United States, initially with non-purified biological preparations containing IL-2 and more recently with RIL-2, in a variety of animal tumour models, have demonstrated the ability of *in vitro* generated LAK cells, in conjuntion with IL-2, to destroy tumour cells leading to substantial regression and/or disappearance of tumour deposits (Foon 1989). The IL-2 and LAK cells appeared not to damage normal tissue elements. Studies carried out, to date, in man using either the intravenous or subcutaneous route have documented a variable beneficial response, the latter being seen in patients with renal cell carcinoma and malignant melanoma (approximately 25 per cent, predominantly partial response). The response rate with the more common tumours, e.g., breast and colon cancer, has been disappointingly low. However, the precise dose, duration of therapy, and route of administration has still to be defined. Toxicity is common, dose-dependent, and a wide spectrum of side-effects have been documented with LAK and RIL-2 therapy. LAK cells are generated by the bulk culturing *in vitro* of blood lymphocytes (previously stimulated *in vivo* with RIL-2) with RIL-2 for three to four days. The blood lymphocytes are isolated from the circulation, using a leucophoresis machine and separated from the remaining white and red blood cells. The generated LAK cells are then re-infused with RIL-2 into the patient. Efficiency of immune modulation by infusion of RIL-2 is monitored by the rebound lymphocytosis and eosinophilia. Another strategy employed is the determination of NK and LAK cells generated by phenotype characterization of cells (e.g. $CD16^+$, $CD56^+$) and *in vitro* killer cell assays. Some recent studies, however, suggest that the complex cytokine cascade, triggered by RIL-2 and LAK cell infusions, may be just as important as the generation of killer cells, in inducing tumour cell death. The advent of IL-2, IFN, TNF, and other cytokines into clinical practice has ushered in a new, exciting, and potentially beneficial form of anti-cancer immunotherapy. Advances have been rapid, but many more careful and well planned trials are needed to evaluate more precisely this new form of treatment. (Foon, 1989)

7.5.2 Non-specific modulators

Microbial agents

For many years bacteria and their various extracts have been used intermittently and with a variable degree of success, to boost host defences, particularly those directed against malignant disease. The most widely used and evaluated in clinical trials in man has been BCG. The rationale for its use was its proven ability to enhance CMI and induce regression of tumours in animal models. Also, it was shown to induce regression of cutaneous tumour deposits (when injected directly into the deposits) in patients with malignant melanoma. Numerous prospective trials, however, using adjuvant BCG following surgery for different types of solid cancers (melanoma, lung, breast), have failed to demonstrate significant survival benefit. When administered locally (pleural cavity, bladder, intra-tumour), on the other hand, significant anti-tumour effects have been demonstrated with an associated influx of lymphoreticular cells. The beneficial effects, however, have tended to be short-lived. When administered with irradiated tumour cells (leukaemic blasts, colonic cancer cells) it can, in a substantial number of patients, induce cutaneous DTH responses to autologous tumour cells. The relevance of these findings to improved clinical survival has yet to be delineated.

Synthetic compounds

In recent years, a number of synthetic compounds, many occurring also as natural molecules, have been produced—polyribonucleotides, muramyl dipeptide, tuftsin, thymosin, levamisole, etc. Studies in animals have documented enhancement of aspects of both humoral and cellular immunity with the various compounds. Based on these findings, a number of these agents have been evaluated in clinical practice, particularly as anti-tumour substances. Levamisole, which had been used as an anti-helminthic, has been shown to effect T cell and monocyte-macrophage function. Its anti-tumour effect in advanced malignancy, both in experimental animals and man, appears to be enhanced if given in conjunction with chemotherapeutic agents. Previously, it has not been shown to be of value when used as an adjuvant following surgery for solid cancers. More recently, preliminary evidence suggest a possible beneficial role in conjunction with 5-FU for colo-rectal cancer. Further studies are needed to evaluate its role in cancer immunotherapy. The synthetic double stranded polyribonucleotides (Poly A: poly U, Poly I: poly C) can enhance both humoral immunity (enhanced antibody production), acting as adjuvant, and CMI, in particular NK cell activity. The polyribonucleotides are inducers of interferon production, which leads to enhancement of NK cell activity, both in man and animals. Studies in women with breast cancer, using Poly A: poly U, show some survival advantage in patients with nodal invasion by tumour. Other studies are in progress, evaluating its effect in patients with melanoma and stomach cancer.

7.6 Miscellaneous

7.6.1 Histamine receptor antagonists

Evidence has accumulated over the past two decades suggesting that histamine plays an important role *in situ* in regulating the inflammatory response and immune reactivity. It is postulated that histamine modulates host defence mechanisms by interacting with histamine (H) receptors (R), which are distributed on surface membranes of T lymphocyte subsets. The evidence for such receptors, in particular H_2R, is based mainly on functional studies. The molecular events, underlying transduction sequences following interaction of histamine and the cell membrane receptors, are being gradually delineated; intracellular cAMP modulation appears to play an important role. In general, by interacting with H_2R, *histamine induces inhibition of lymphocyte reactivity*, either directly or through the release *in situ* of suppressor factors (e.g., prostaglandins) possibly by T lymphocytes. Histamine has been shown to inhibit lymphocyte reactivity to mitogens and alloantigens (in both man and animals) and DTH responses of skin to topical agents. It suppresses the release of cytokines—IL-2, IFN,—but the effects are variable and dependent on the methodology used. It inhibits to a variable degree, *in vitro* cellular cytotoxicity (T cell, K and NK cell-mediated) although some studies have shown it to enhance effector-target cell interactivity and enhance K and NK cell activity. Lastly, it down-regulates the production of antibodies in response to antigens, probably by suppression of T helper cell activity.

H_2R antagonists (Cimetidine, Ranitidine) are used extensively in medical practice. In recent years, H_2R-blockers have been prescribed, with increasing frequency, to traumatized patients, particularly in intensive care units, and to certain high-risk groups in the peri-operative period, to minimize or prevent the occurrence of bleeding from stress-induced ulcers and gastric erosions. Cimetidine and Ranitidine have been shown to have pronounced effects on various aspects of the immune response, both in man and experimental animals. These modulations of immune reactivity have been demonstrated in different *in vitro* assays and documented following therapy with these drugs. *H_2R antagonists* effect these changes predominantly by *blocking the action of histamine* and in particular its effect on the release of various *suppressive factors by mononuclear cells*. The enhancing effects of Cimetidine have been seen primarily in those clinical situations and experimental models where inhibition or defects of immune reactivity were probably due to excessive and/or prolonged activity of T suppressor cells (and possibly macrophages). Therapy with Cimetidine has been shown: (1) to prevent the alterations in the circulating levels of $CD4^+$ and $CD8^+$ cells that occur following major surgery; (2) to prevent the depression of DTH responses in man, induced by peri-operative blood transfusions; (3) to enhance NK cell activity (*in vitro* and *in vivo*) in patients with low levels of cytotoxicity (leukaemias and solid tumours); and (4) to augment the secretion of immunoglobulin and antibodies in patients with variable hypogammoglobulinaemia. Preliminary studies have shown an apparent beneficial effect in reducing tumour load both in animals and man, particularly when Cimetidine was used with other cytotoxic or immunostimulatory drugs. These various results must be interpreted with caution and more detailed studies need to be carried out to evaluate these non-traditional roles of H_2R antagonists, if any, in clinical practice.

7.6.2 Oestrogen receptor antagonists

Many patients with clinically localized breast cancer, (but with suspected occult metastases), receive systemic adjuvant therapy (Tamoxifen) for prolonged periods of time following surgery. Studies with small numbers of such women suggest that Tamoxifen may enhance NK cell activity, both increased numbers of $CD16^+$ cells as well as enhanced *in vitro* cytotoxicity have been demonstrated. Further sequential studies are needed to define continued NK cell activity with prolonged therapy and its clinical relevance to survival.

References and Further reading

Collins, J.A. (1989). Current status of blood therapy in surgery. *Advances in Surgery*, **22**, 75–104.

Foon, K.A. Biological response modifiers: The new immunotherapy. *Cancer Research*, **49**, 1621–39.

Stevenson, G.W., Hall, S.C., Rudwick, S., Seleny, F.L., and Stevenson, H.C., (1990). The effect of anaesthetic agents on the human immune response (Review). *Anaesthesiology*, **72**, 542–52.

8
Autoimmune disease, human immunodeficiency virus (HIV) infection, and the surgeon

H.F. Sewell

8.1 Introduction

Autoimmune reactions, characterized by the presence of autoantibodies and autoreactive T cells, can be demonstrated in a significant number of diseases. In some situations, such as following surgery, trauma, and infection, the autoreactive elements appear to be transient and of little clinico-pathological relevance. Contrastingly, many major rheumatological, endocrinological, haematological, and liver disorders (see Table 8.1) have autoimmune reactions which are clearly of major significance in the pathophysiology of the clinical disorders. In this chapter limited aspects of autoimmune diseases are presented in a didactic manner, and are not meant to be exhaustive, but rather to be of direct clinical usefulness to specialist surgical practice. For further clinical details see Chapel and Haeney, (1988). Considerations of the aetiology of autoimmune disease and practical assays used to evaluate autoimmunity can be found respectively in Chapters 1 and 9.

The numbers of cases of AIDS and of HIV infection, as documented by the World Health Organization (WHO), continue to rise at striking rates

Table 8.1. The autoimmune disease spectrum

Organ specific	MIXED SPECIFICITY		**Non-organ specific**
Graves' Disease	Myasthenia gravis	Primary biliary cirrhosis	Rheumatoid arthritis (RA)
Chronic thyroiditis			Systemic lupus erythematosus (SLE)
	Goodpasture's syndrome	Autoimmune chronic active hepatitis	
Autoimmune gastritis			Discoid lupus erythematosus
Pernicious anaemia	Autoimmune uveitis	Autoimmune heamolytic anaemia	Other connective tissue diseases (CTD)
Diabetes mellitus (type 1)—insulin-dependent	Pemphigus vulgaris pemphigoid	Autoimmune thrombocytopaenic purpura	Sjögren's syndrome; most cases are of secondary type, associated with RA, SLE, and other CTDs
Addison's disease			
Sjögren's syndrome (SS); a few cases of primary SS			
Autoimmunity to: Spermatozoa, Ovarian antigens	Sympathetic ophthalmia		

in many parts of the world. It is likely that most of us in medical practice will or have encountered patients infected with the human immunodeficiency virus. An overview of AIDS and HIV infection is presented together with consideration of their impact on surgical practice.

A AUTOIMMUNE DISEASE AND THE SURGEON

8.2 Organ specific autoimmunity (OSA)

OSA exists in conditions where tolerance to self antigens (which are expressed by and restricted to a particular organ) is abrogated, and autoantibodies and autoreactive T cells can be demonstrated. In this situation of abnormal immune regulation the autoreactive components in some cases can be shown to cause direct tissue damage and are termed *primary* agents. In other cases they appear to be *secondary*, and arise as a consequence of tissue damage. In clinical practice, most of the evidence indicates that autoantibodies are of crucial importance in the induction of tissue-damaging reactions and, accordingly, most emphasis is directed to measuring autoantibodies rather than autoreactive T cells. OSA is largely associated with endocrinopathy (Table 8.1) and autoantibodies can be demonstrated against endocrine cells, their products or the hormone receptors on target tissues. Measurement of these autoantibodies can prove useful in establishing the diagnosis and in monitoring disease activity and response to therapy.

8.2.1 Thyroid autoimmunity

Antibodies have been established as the primary agents in *Graves' disease*. These have been shown to be IgG autoantibodies, directed against the thyroid-stimulating hormone (TSH) receptor on the thyroid epithelial cells. Their interaction with the TSH receptor results in the continuous stimulation of the gland and in excess production of tri-iodo thyronine (T3) and thyroxine (T4), as well as stimulation of the growth of the gland and production of a goitre. Other autoreactive T cells and antibodies have been shown to bind to retro-orbital antigens and to contribute to the exophthalmos. Previously termed long-acting thyroid stimulator (LATS), the IgG anti-TSH receptor autoantibody is generally not measured when diagnosing Graves' disease.

Chronic thyroiditis

Testing for autoantibodies can be helpful in diagnosing autoimmune thyroiditis (Hashimoto's disease) in patients presenting with a goitre and in a euthyroid state. The two most useful antibodies to measure are *anti-thyroglobulin* (anti-T: directed to the macromolecular protein of the colloid), and *anti-microsome* (anti-M: directed to the cytosolic microsomes found within the thyroid epithelial cells surrounding the colloid). Both antibody tests should be requested, as together they give a high diagnostic yield. One or both autoantibodies are significantly increased in autoimmune thyroid disease compared to other causes of a goitre, where very low levels of the antibodies may be recorded. Anti-T and anti-M are classically thought of as 'secondary' autoantibodies which arise due to thyroid tissue damage. The gland can be shown to be infiltrated with $CD8^+$ T cells together with B lymphocytes, plasma cells, and macrophages. The chronic thyroiditis patients who may require surgery for cosmetic or other reasons and have high levels (titres) of anti-M are believed to be likely to eventually develop significant thyroid hypofunction. Accordingly, such information (i.e., anti-M titre) may be one important factor for the surgeon to consider with regard to the degree of thyroid resection undertaken.

In obstetric practice, cases of *transient post-partum hypothyroidism*, usually presenting within six months of delivery, are associated with increased levels of anti-T and anti-M antibodies. Most women improve spontaneously but evidence indicates that those with high levels of anti-M are unlikely to go into remission.

8.2.2 Gastric autoimmunity and pernicious anaemia

Gastritis associated with low acid production, high serum gastrin levels and with autoantibodies to *gastric parietal cells* and *intrinsic factor* is associated with pernicious anaemia, and is believed to be autoimmune in origin. Patients with autoimmune gastritis also commonly have thyroid autoantibodies (anti-T and anti-M), although they are most often euthyroid. A similar finding is obtained for patients with chronic thyroiditis. This accords with the general finding that patients with a clinically expressed OSA disorder can have autoantibodies to other organs without clinical disease in that organ. These patients commonly have a family history of such disorders.

Pernicious anaemia (PA), which has no specific clinical picture can present with a sore tongue (>25 per cent of cases), general tiredness (>90 per cent), or with the much more serious neurological features of subacute combined degeneration of the spinal cord (<5 per cent of cases). A useful immunological assay is the measurement of parietal cell antibodies (parietal cell antibodies: positive in over 90 per cent of patients), although it is of low specificity. Parietal cell antibodies are found in from 2 to 20 per cent of the aged population, in iron deficiency anaemia, and in association with other autoimmune disorders; thus it is best seen as a clinical screening test. Intrinsic factor antibodies, although less sensitive (positive in 50 to 80 per cent of patients), is much more specific for PA and is an extremely useful diagnostic test. Intrinsic factor antibodies rarely occurs without overt or latent PA. Measurement of parietal cell antibodies and intrinsic factor antibodies are especially useful and non-invasive procedures when the Schilling test is equivocal.

8.3 Non-organ specific autoimmunity

In these disorders autoantibodies and autoreactive T cells can be demonstrated with specificity for antigens which are distributed widely throughout various organs and tissues. The antigens are usually subcellular particles or membrane-associated and may be secreted into the circulation. Many of the listed non-organ specific autoimmune diseases (see Table 8.1) show elements of abnormal immunological activity and regulation (Chapter 1, Section 1.6.2). The autoantibodies detected are commonly helpful in diagnosis and prognosis, although their ability to define the tissues involved and their role in the aetiology of the disorder are far from clear.

8.3.1 Rheumatoid arthritis (RA)

This affects approximately 1 per cent of the adult population and can present at any age and involve any joint. Some extra-articular manifestations, which may present to surgeons in various specialities without the classic joint and X-ray stigmata, should be borne in mind. Thus, chronic skin ulcers, carpel tunnel syndrome, episcleritis, oral ulcers, nerve root compressions, and lymphadenopathy may all be associated with and should raise the clinical suspicion of a diagnosis of RA. Immune serology can be an aid to diagnosis, and of value in prognosis. Rheumatoid factor (RF) is classically an IgM autoantibody directed to the patient's own IgG immunoglobulin. This classic RF is detected in approximately 80 per cent of RA patients, especially those with more aggressive disease (the so-called seropositive RAs). Twenty per cent of patients lack classical RF (seronegative RA) although sophisticated laboratory tests have documented IgG and IgA RF in many 'seronegative RAs'. Classic RF is demonstrated in tests such as the 'Rose–Waaler', which uses the patient's serum containing RF to agglutinate indicator red blood cells coated with IgG immunoglobulin. RF can also be demonstrated in synovial joint fluid and may contribute to local tissue damage by activating complement and stimulating inflammatory cell migration and activation. The production of cytokines, such as IL-1, IL-2, and IL-6, may also contribute to the tissue damage. Currently, the measurement of RF is seen as a prognostic indicator, whereby high levels correlate with more severe and progressive disease, but it remains a poor indicator in monitoring disease activity or the efficacy of therapy; to that end the measurement of C-reactive protein (CRP) is much more useful, even more so than ESR.

8.3.2 Seronegative arthritides

These exclude those cases associated with known infections, and are characterized by the absence of all RFs in the serum. They include conditions, such as ankylosing spondylitis (AS), psoriatic and enteropathic arthritis, Reiters' and Behçet's syndromes, and rarer disorders such as relapsing polychondritis. The latter three conditions may present varyingly to eye, ENT and dental/oral surgeons, and some of the former to the orthopaedic surgeon. Currently, there are no immunological tests of sufficient sensitivity or specificity that contribute meaningfully to clinical diagnosis, with the possible exception of typing for the HLA-B27 antigen in suspected cases of AS. The association of HLA-B27 with AS is very strong (see Chapter 1, Section 1.3.1, MHC antigens) and its occurrence in the Caucasian non-AS population is low. Thus, in a suspected case of AS the *absence of HLA-B27 makes the diagnosis very unlikely.*

8.3.3 Paediatric chronic arthritis

In the investigation of chronic arthritis in children which may be due to many disorders, including infections, juvenile RA (JRA), juvenile AS (JAS), and the varying forms of juvenile chronic arthritis (JCA), the paediatric physician and surgeon should find the measurement of rheumatoid factor and anti-nuclear autoantibodies (ANA) particularly useful. The JCA grouping-classification of some authorities include cases of JRA (~10 per cent) which behave like adult RA and the presence of RF confirms the diagnosis. Such children have a form of RA which tends to progress to severe joint destruction and have associated extra-articular complications, such as vasculitis. Early diagnosis contributes to more efficient clinical management. JAS (~15 per cent of cases) behaves similarly to the adult disease and the association of and testing for the HLA-B27 antigen is equally relevant. The remaining forms of JCA include the systemic disorder (synonymous with Still's disease), the pauciarticular and the polyarticular disease. Children in the pauciarticular grouping who have a positive ANA appear to have a greatly increased risk of developing chronic iridocyclitis. The measurement of CRP also proves useful in the monitoring of disease activity in cases of childhood non-infection associated arthritis.

8.3.4 Systemic lupus erythematosus (SLE)

This is the prototype non-organ specific autoimmune disorder which is associated with anti-nuclear autoantibodies (ANA) and more specifically with antibodies to double stranded (native) DNA. The latter represent the two most definitive laboratory assays for the diagnosis of SLE. Lupus has protean manifestations and can present to any medical or surgical speciality.

Table 8.2. Clinical presentation and cumulative organ pathology in SLE

Clinical presentation	%	**Organ involvement**	%
Arthritis/arthralgia	62	Joint/muscle	98
Skin lesions	~20	Skin	98
Thrombocytopaenic purpura and haemolytic anaemia Recurrent thrombophlebitis	~10	Blood	60
Neuropsychiatric problems	~4–5	Brain	60
		Kidney	40
		Heart	20

The multi-systemic nature of SLE, which typically affects young females, is shown with respect to presenting features and organ involvement in Table 8.2.

Table 8.2 reveals that skin involvement is frequent in SLE, and a biopsy can be diagnostic. Immunofluorescent staining of frozen sections shows granular deposits of immunoglobulins and complement components at the epidermal–dermal junction (the lupus band test). In excess of 70 per cent of SLE patients have a 'positive' skin biopsy test.

SLE activity is evaluated by the sequential monitoring of the serum levels of complement components C3 and C4 and other complement breakdown-activation products. With active disease and substantial organ involvement C3 and C4 are detected at subnormal levels due to their consumption by immune complexes (antigens and autoantibodies) and activation of the complement system (see Chapter 1, Section 1.5.1). With diminished disease activity the C3 and C4 serum levels return toward the normal range. The levels of complement products are more sensitive than the ESR, or sequential ANA or DNA antibody levels in monitoring disease activity.

Recent clinical assays of 'free' CD25 antigen (the IL-2 receptor) in blood and other body fluids suggests that it is a good marker of immune activation and should prove useful in the monitoring of disease activity in SLE and RA.

8.4 Overview of autoantibodies in clinical practice

Organ specific and non-organ specific autoimmune diseases are often presented as two distinct groups, but in reality the clinical and laboratory evidence indicate that they are part of a spectrum of autoimmune disorders (see Table 8.1). Table 8.3 summarizes a selection of autoantibody tests which may prove useful in varying aspects of surgical practice. For example, a fairly rapid onset of ascites and deepening jaundice is one of the presentations of primary biliary cirrhosis (PBC). The findings of high serum levels

Table 8.3. Tests for autoantibodies*

Test	Normal range	Report	Interpretation
Anti-nuclear antibody (ANA)	Negative (but <1/20 titre IgG often found in 'normals')	1. Negative or Positive 2. Titre IgG class 3. Staining pattern	Negative ANA virtually excludes SLE. Speckled ANA suggestive of mixed connective tissue disease. Nucleolar ANA suggestive of scleroderma.
Anti-centromere antibodies	Negative	Negative or Positive	Suggestive of scleroderma especially the CREST varient. Many patients present with idiopathic Raynauds.
Anti-Ro (SS-A) antibodies (Ro/La small protein antigens found in the nucleus and cytoplasm of cells)	Negative	Negative or Positive	1. Especially useful in SLE presenting with prominent photosensitive cutaneous lupus. 2. Ro positive lupus have been described in the ANA negative SLE groups. 3. Anti-Ro—useful in the investigation of patients with a history of recurrent spontaneous miscarriage.
Anti-La (SS-B) antibodies	Negative	Negative or Positive	Positive in 10% of SLE. La antibodies usually found together with Ro antibodies. Ro and La antibodies have been found in almost all mothers and infants with neonatal lupus syndrome.

Rheumatoid factor (RF)	Units and normal ranges will be quoted by laboratorires with respect to their system of analysis		Useful in differential diagnosis of connective tissue disorders.
Anti-mitochondrial antibodies (AMA)	Negative	1. Negative or Positive 2. Titre	Strong positive associated with primary biliary cirrhosis.
Anti-phospholipid and Anti-cardiolipin antibodies	Determined by the laboratory	Positive 1+ to 3+ or ELISA units	Associated with thrombotic disease – small and large vessels. - As part of SLE syndrome with the lupus anti-coagulant. - A discrete phospholipid syndrome.
Anti-smooth muscle antibodies (SMA)	Negative (but SMA, of low positivity often found with viral infection)	1. Negative or Positive 2. Grade 1+ to 3+	Strong positive associated with chronic active hepatitis.
Anti-thyroid antibody Anti-thyroglobulin	Less than 1/20	1. Titre	Useful in the differential diagnosis of a goitre.
Anti-microsomal antibodies	Less than 1/100 (different laboratories will quote their established normal ranges)	2. Titre	High titre: found in over 90% of cases of autoimmune thyroiditis. Low titre: found in 30% of Graves' disease and about 10% of adenocarcinomas.
Gastric parietal cell (GPC) antibodies	Negative	1. Negative or Positive 2. Grade 1+ to 3+	Associated with atrophic gastritis – found in >90% of cases of PA and 40% of cases of gastric atrophy. Found in 30% of patients with autoimmune thyroid disease. GPC antibodies may be the first indication of an autoimmune organ specific disorder, e.g., in the investigation of a macrocytosis.

Table 8.3. cont'd

Test	Normal range	Report	Interpretation
Intrinsic factor antibody	Negative	Negative or Positive	Occurs in >70% of pernicious anaemia cases. More specific for PA than GPC antibodies.
Skin antibodies Epidermal (basement membrane) Intercellular cement (desmosomal)	Negative	Negative or Positive	Useful in the differential diagnosis of bullous eruptions.
Antibodies to adrenal cortex (adrenal antibody)	Negative	Negative or Positive	Positive in about 65% of cases of idiopathic adrenal insufficiency.
Skeletal muscle antibody	Negative	Negative or Positive	Found in 40–50% of myasthenia gravis. Anti-acetylcholine receptor antibody more sensitive and specific.
Neutrophil antibody (NA)	Negative	Negative or Positive	Very useful in differential diagnosis of vasculitides – NA positive in Wegener's, microscopic polyarteritis, and related disorders.

* The autoantibodies listed have varying degrees of clinical usefulness and discriminatory value in diagnosis and management. Information should be obtained by discussion with the consultant immunologist or other trained specialist personnel regarding uncertainty about tests, their interpretation, and values.

of anti-mitochondrial autoantibody together with high levels of serum IgM (~80 per cent of cases) rapidly establishes the diagnosis of PBC. Consultation with a clinical immunologist or other relevant personnel should ensure the most efficacious use of such investigations.

B HUMAN IMMUNODEFICIENCY VIRUS (HIV), ACQUIRED IMMUNODEFICIENCY SYNDROME (AIDS), AND THE SURGEON

8.5 AIDS and HIV

8.5.1 Aetiopathology

The AIDS pandemic was first recognized in 1981 when a group of men presented with rare opportunistic infections and tumours which were indicative of an underlying cellular immune deficiency, but without any obvious cause for such a deficiency. That clinical definition of the syndrome was followed in 1983 by the discovery of the retrovirus, now called HIV, which is known to be the central agent in the aetiopathology of AIDS. (Retroviruses contain the unique enzyme reverse transcriptase (RT) which allows them to copy their RNA → proviral DNA, the 'reversal' of the normal flow of genetic events). The delineation of the prototype HIV-1 has been followed by the isolation of another member of the *Lentivirus* grouping termed HIV-2 which is also capable of causing AIDS. Distantly related retroviruses have also been isolated from several monkey species and are named simian immunodeficiency virus (SIV).

Figure 8.1 shows the overall organizational structure of HIV together with some of the detectable antibodies to viral proteins (antigens) found in infected people. Figure 8.2 shows some of the clinical manifestations of AIDS. In the West, most AIDS patients have presented with opportunistic infections, especially prominent being *pneumocystis carinii* pneumonitis (in excess of 60 per cent of cases) and Kaposi's sarcoma. Other infections with pathogenic and opportunistic bacteria, viruses, protozoa, and fungi also cause havoc in such patients with a deficient immune system.

AIDS patients in certain parts of the world (e.g., Africa), with a differing spectrum of environmental microflora, have differing patterns of clinical presentation. In parts of Africa, AIDS patients often present with severe malabsorption and a wasting syndrome (called Slim's disease) together with disseminated infections, such as tuberculosis.

8.5.2 Epidemiology and transmission of HIV infection

AIDS represents only the end-stage manifestation of infection, which may take many years to develop following initial infection with HIV. It is

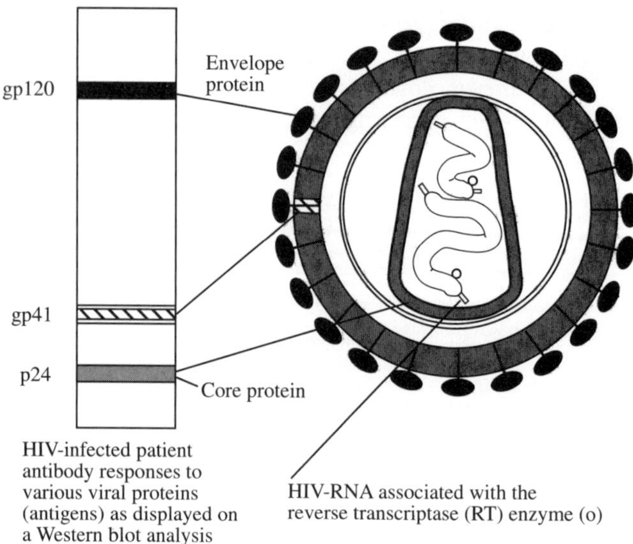

Fig. 8.1. Scheme of the organization of the HIV-1 retrovirus.

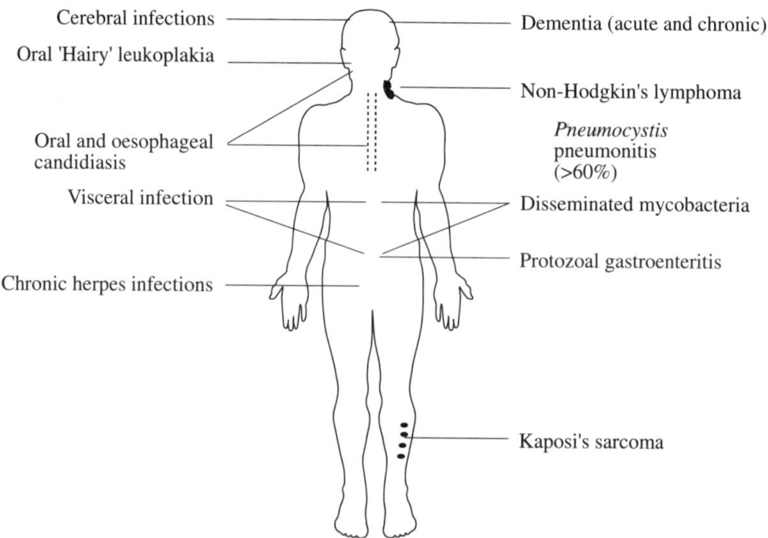

Fig. 8.2. AIDS—some clinical associations/manifestations. (1) The agents associated with AIDS pathology: involves opportunistic infection (protozoal, fungal, bacterial, and viral) together with well-known pathogens. (2) Neuropathological disorders are well recognized without concomitant infections. (3) Associated tumours are being increasingly recognized, beyond the well-documented Kaposi's sarcoma.

commonly estimated that for every documented case of AIDS there may be 20–30 times as many HIV infected persons. By mid-1991 the WHO global programme on AIDS had documented in excess of 350 000 cases of AIDS. Due to under-recognition/diagnosis and under-reporting of cases, especially in developing countries, the WHO believes that the true figures are in excess of 500 000. Currently, the WHO estimates that there are in excess of 10 million HIV infected people world-wide.

HIV-infected persons may be asymptomatic or present with a spectrum of clinical manifestations, including those associated with AIDS. Various attempts are made to classify and stage the spectrum of HIV infection. Figure 8.3 shows some of the recognized features/stages of HIV infection correlated with time and measureable immunological indices.

Epidemiological studies have clearly documented the means of spread of the infection (Adler, 1987), which are:

Sexual intercourse
- Anal and vaginal

Needle route
- Intravenous drug abuse
- 'Needlestick' injuries
- Injections

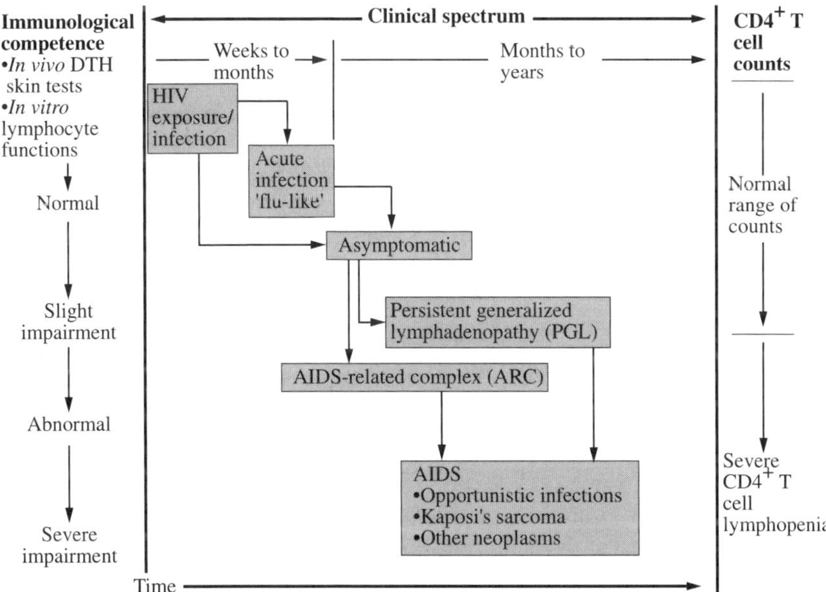

Fig. 8.3. Progression of HIV infection to AIDS. Correlates of clinical spectrum, immunological competence, and $CD4^+$ T cell counts with time.

Mother and child
- *In utero* (vertical transmission)
- Perinatal
- Breast milk

Tissues and organs for transplantation
- Blood
- Kidneys
- Skin, bone marrow, etc.

Recognition of the means of viral transmission accordingly indicates some of the means of prevention. It is axiomatic that prevention is better than cure, but, today, with this particular viral infection *prevention is the only cure*. Current policies, national and world-wide, are directed to prevention strategies involving education—to overcome public ignorance, to teach safe sex, and to change behaviour. There is also substantial funding for biomedical research aimed at developing suitable pharmaceuticals, vaccines, and other treatment modalities against HIV infection. The recent outstanding scientific advances in molecular and cell biology have led to a better understanding of the nature of the virus and its interaction with the host cells. This knowledge has highlighted the major difficulties which are present and will be encountered in trying to find an effective therapy or vaccine for HIV. It has also, however, revealed possible weaknesses in the viral 'armour' which could be breached.

8.5.3 Immunology of AIDS and HIV

The pathology and clinical features of HIV infection and AIDS can be understood in terms of the immunology of HIV-host interaction. The virus targets the $CD4^+$ cells, especially the helper/inducer T lymphocytes, the central cell of the immune response (see Chapter 1, Section 1.3.3). The HIV gp120 outer coat molecule (see Fig. 8.1) uses the CD4 molecule on the T cell as its receptor. The initial binding of HIV to the CD4 molecule is the major prerequisite for infection. Following fusion of HIV to the T cell membrane a series of events ensue. The retrovirus, having entered the host cell, uses its RT directed and newly synthesized proviral DNA form and certain enzymes to intergrate into the host genomic DNA. It then uses the cell's 'hijacked' genetic apparatus to make new viruses. Thus, HIV incorporates itself into the $CD4^+$ T cell, and into any other cell which expresses the CD4 receptor molecule—macrophages, monocytes, Langerhans cells of skin, and other antigen-presenting cells (APCs); and some cells of the central nervous system, such as glial cells. Each of these cell types have been demonstrated to be sites of harbouring, incorporation, and expression of HIV.

Infected $CD4^+$ T cells, in time, malfunction and/or are destroyed by a series of, as yet, incompletely defined mechanisms. The latter include direct viral toxic effects, and the probable induction of indirect destructive 'autoimmune reactions'-autoantibodies and autoreactive cytotoxic cells. Over months to years a decline in $CD4^+$ T cells can be measured, and in fact it is one of the important prognostic monitors of progression of HIV infection towards AIDS (see Fig. 8.3). Many factors involved in the progression of HIV infection to AIDS are as yet ill-defined. As explained in Chapter 1, $CD4^+$ T cells are important *regulators* and *effector* cells in the immune response and are the effectors of cell-mediated immune (CMI) reactions which protect against intracellular infections and the development of tumours. Accordingly, many of the opportunistic and pathogenic infections, and tumours seen in HIV infection/AIDS, can be attributed to loss or functional impairment of the critical $CD4^+$ cells. Other associations of HIV infection, such as dementia and neuropathies, are not so readily explained and can be encountered in patients with normal numbers and functional $CD4^+$ T cells. The genesis of AIDS-associated Kaposi's sarcoma appears to involve deregulated cytokine growth factor(s) stimulation of the target endothelial cells rather than a direct HIV infection-associated pathology.

8.5.4 Serum antibodies in AIDS and HIV infection

The serum antibodies detected in HIV-infected people (see Fig. 8.1) are believed, in the main, to be non-protective with regard to the natural history and progression to AIDS. Current evidence indicates that the majority of HIV-infected individuals will have progressive disease, probably over many years (without therapeutic intervention). The laboratory tests designed to detect antibodies, e.g., anti-gp120, anti-gp41, and anti-p24 have been extremely useful for documenting HIV status, for screening blood and organ donors, and for epidemiological studies. The antibody test also indicates that following exposure to the virus, there is a period of several weeks during which the individual is probably infectious (HIV can be cultured from infected lymphocytes and p24 antigen can be found in blood) before antibody is detectable. Thus, amongst the many social, legal, economic, and medical arguments concerning the advantages and disadvantages of antibody screening for HIV status, it must be clearly understood that the antibody tests, though exceedingly useful, are unreliable in the early stages of infection.

8.5.5 AIDS and HIV infection, and surgical practice

Surgeons realize that there is a growing number of people in the community infected by HIV, some of whom will undoubtedly become patients under their care. Some will be known to be HIV infected or have AIDS and may require surgical treatment, or invasive investigations. Others will present as patients with a normal spectrum of surgical problems, unrelated to their HIV status. Thus, the question must be asked as to whether surgeons are at high occupational risk and if so what can be done to mitigate such risk. Blood and blood products are a major source of transmission of the virus and are of course constantly in the working arena of surgeons. Surveys show surgeons inflicting self-injury with needles or knives (to the order of 15–20 per cent) in the course of their duties; glove puncture occurs in up to one-quarter to one-third of operations. Although the risk of virus transmission appears potentially high, the number of recorded cases of surgeons becoming infected with HIV, as with other health care personnel, is very low. Perhaps this might change for the worse if current practices continue and HIV infection in the community continues to increase. What then should surgeons do? What special precautions or measures should be taken? The following comments are those personally held by the author, some of which are supported by current national guidelines. Readers should refer to international and UK Health Department guidelines (see suggested reading).

1. *Known AIDS/HIV infected patient.* Adopt similar precautions to those recommended for patients who are hepatitis B virus antigen positive. Some surgical units in the United States with *a significant community* of HIV positive individuals assume all patients carry the virus. That may well represent extreme caution, but it should remind all those in medical/paramedical practice to treat human blood with the necessary caution.

2. *High-risk groups.* If the patient is known to indulge in 'risky' practices (sex with prostitutes/promiscuous sex, homosexual practices, drug abusers/addicts), either currently or previously, then surgery should be performed assuming that the patient is infected with HIV. To require compulsory HIV testing of the patient prior to surgery, involves many legal and ethical dilemmas. Even if a patient in such a high-risk group was found on testing to be HIV antibody negative, that could never be taken as an absolute guarantee of not being infected with the virus and, therefore, not infectious.

3. *Donors.* Donors of *all* organs and semen should be screened for the presence of HIV antibody in blood and, more importantly, potential donors should be made aware of high-risk groups. If they fall into any of the known categories (homosexuals, drug abusers, prostitutes, etc.) they, like blood donors, should desist from donation.

4. *HIV has been isolated from* plasma, leucocytes, semen, cervical secretions, breast milk, tears, saliva, urine, and cerebrospinal fluid. There is considerable doubt that infection is transmitted from the latter four fluids.

If body fluids (from known HIV-positive patients) are spilled on skin, eyes, or other mucous membranes, these should be washed immediately with copious amounts of fluid.

5. *Penetrating wounds* ('needlestick,' scalpel) should be encouraged to bleed, and I would advocate washing with 70 per cent ethanol/isopropyl alcohol or phenolics (which are known to kill the virus). Even in the light of the very few seroconversions documented for 'needlestick' injuries with known HIV positive blood, I think in these circumstances and for larger penetrating wounds, having followed the suggestions above, I would advise that a short course (14–28 days) of the anti-viral agent AZT/Zidovudine 200 mg/4 h (see below) be given, commencing within 24 hours of the injury. The injury should be reported to the appropriate medical personnel, and a sample of blood taken and stored for comparison with future follow-up samples. With time and experience these may be modified.

Guidelines concerning the spillage of HIV infected blood, decontamination of equipment, and protocols for the control of infection, are clearly documented in several WHO circulars and in several DHSS publications in the United Kingdom.

8.5.6 Anti-viral therapy and strategies

Currently, the only recommended drug for clinical use with proven anti-HIV activity, albeit very limited, is the nucleoside analogue 3′azido-3′-deoxythymidine (Zidovudine—formerly azidothymidine, AZT). (Henderson and Gerberding, 1989). Zidovudine attacks one of the weak points in the HIV armoury. The viral enzyme RT, which uses the viral RNA as a template to synthesize DNA, is unique to the virus and is not present in man. RT uses the human nucleotide thymidine as one of the building blocks in making up the viral DNA chain. HIV/RT will also use the analogue of thymidine, i.e. AZT/Zidovudine just as readily. When AZT is incorporated into the growing viral DNA chain, it prevents the addition of other human nucleoside building blocks which are not compatible, thus resulting in the termination in DNA chain synthesis, which is expressed as inhibition of viral replication.

Double-blind clinical trials, initially performed in the United States, demonstrated that AZT prolongs the life, albeit for short periods, of certain subgroups of AIDS patients and diminishes the frequency of associated pneumonia. Currently, studies are underway to examine the efficacy of AZT in asymptomatic, HIV-infected (non-AIDS) patients.

There are formidable problems associated with the use of the drug AZT. First, with the necessary long-term use (all evidence indicates that when the drug is stopped in AIDS patients, viral replication recommences) toxic effects can occur, especially on bone marrow haematopoiesis. Some patients become dependent on repeated transfusions. Other experimental nucleoside analogues have resulted in patients developing severe neuropathies. Furthermore, recent laboratory data has indicated that long-term treatment with AZT results in the emergence of drug resistant strains (mutations) of HIV. Whether such mutants will prove damaging clinically is uncertain, but clearly it is a worrying prospect, especially if AZT is to be used in HIV-infected but asymptomatic individuals over long periods.

One promising therapeutic approach is directed against the initial and critical reaction of the HIV envelope protein gp120 with the CD4 receptor on T cells. Several research groups are using soluble forms of recombinant DNA-derived CD4, and modified CD4 to bind to the viral protein in order to block viral binding to and infection of T lymphocytes. Non-cell associated HIV is a very fragile and vulnerable virus. Clinical trials based on this approach are in the process of being performed.

Whatever anti-viral therapies eventually prove most beneficial, they will need to be introduced early in the course of the patient's infection, before the virus causes irreversible damage to the immune system. Indeed, anti-viral therapy may need to be combined with immune enhancing manœuvres, such as the use of recombinant cytokines, and bone marrow and thymic transplantation.

8.5.7 Vaccination—prospects

Vaccination approaches are proving much more difficult than anticipated. The use of attenuated viruses, such as in the very effective poliomyelitis vaccine, is not seen as a suitable approach against HIV infection. The virus is known to have a significant mutational ability. Killed HIV has been shown in animals (primate studies) to evoke very poor immune responses, with respect to neutralizing antibodies and cytotoxic cells. Many attempts are being made, using recombinant DNA-derived viral products and novel adjuvants (see Chapter 1), to improve the immunogenicity/antigenicity of HIV products. Some animal experiments have shown that even when 'high' levels of antibody can be induced experimentally, upon challenge with 'wild' HIV, infection is not prevented. Other researchers believe that cytotoxic T cells and other CMI responses may be more important for an effective vaccine. Thus, strategies are being adopted to define viral epitopes and antigens which may induce a significant anti-HIV CMI. Quite likely the best vaccine will be one which induces both significant humoral and CMI against HIV.

The unprecedented effort and co-ordination of biomedical research into finding effective therapies for HIV infection and AIDS gives cause for optimism, although it may take considerable time to be realized. The difficulties involved should not be underestimated nor the hopes overstated.

References and Further reading

Adler, M.W. (ed.) 1987. ABC of AIDS. *British Medical Journal*, **294**.

Chapel, H. and Haeney, M. (1988). Autoimmune diseases in *Essentials of clinical immunology* (2nd edn). Blackwell, Oxford.

Henderson, D.K. and Gerberding, J.L. (1989). Prophylactic Zidovudine after occupational exposure to the human immunodeficiency virus: An interim analysis, *Journal of Infectious Diseases* **160**, 321.

UK Health Department (1990). Guidance for clinical health care workers: protection against HIV and hepatitis viruses: recommendations of the expert advisory group on AIDS. UK Health Department. HMSO, London.

9

Principles of immunological assays and recombinant DNA technology

H.F. Sewell and A. Thomson

9.1 Introduction

Immunological assays have proved extremely useful in patient management and clinical research. Surgeons should have a working knowledge of the principles of the standard assays and of newer developments which may contribute to the scientific understanding of surgery. Outlined below are selected immunological assays together with aspects of modern cellular and recombinant DNA technologies.

9.2 Tumour markers

Cancer is essentially a genetic disorder caused by multi-stage events associated with environmental insults and with changes within the cell which ultimately contribute to the emergence of the cancer phenotype (see Chapter 3). This phenotype differs from normal cellular counterparts by the possession of either unique tumour-specific antigens (TSA), or more commonly, by aberrant expression of normal gene products—differentiation and functional molecules, which are termed tumour-associated antigens (TAA). The increased expression of or secretion of TAA by tumour cells can be detected by immunological assays.

A wide range of monoclonal (and some polyclonal) antibodies have been generated with defined specificity for tumour-associated markers. Their reaction with TSA or TAA are revealed by various detection systems, including immunohistochemical (immunocytochemical) methods, on tissue sections, smears and cells in suspension, and by solid and fluid phase assays such as enzyme-linked immunosorbent assays (ELISA) and radio-immunoassays (RIA).

The immunological assays to be described are used to establish a diagnosis of cancer and to predict prognosis, as well as to monitor the response to therapy in patients with malignant disease.

9.2.1 Principles of techniques and monoclonal antibodies (MABs)

Köhler and Milstein in 1975 described the method of generating potentially limitless quantities of highly specific antibodies to antigens of choice, by fusing *in vitro* an antibody-secreting B cell (to provide specificity of the antibody) with a cultured malignant B cell line (to provide continuous production of antibody) to produce an antibody-secreting, "immortalized" hybridoma. The latter was grown in selective medium, able to support the growth of hybrid cells but not the unfused lymphocytes or tumour cells. Their hybridization method has been employed by various workers to generate numerous MABs with specificity to many TAAs (see Fig. 9.1). (see Chapel and Gooi 1990, for further details). MABs have exquisite specificity as they react with only a single antigenic determinant (an epitope) of complex antigens.

9.2.2 Immunohistochemical techniques

Various sensitive detection systems are employed to demonstrate (visualize) the binding of monoclonal (or polyclonal) antibodies to tumour antigens. The techniques are known by many acronyms such as PAP (peroxidase-antigen-peroxidase), APAAP (alkaline phosphatase–anti-alkaline phosphatase), IFA (indirect fluorescent antibody), and ABC (Avidin–Biotin complex). The principles of these techniques are illustrated in Fig. 9.2. Substrates containing tumour cells or extracts (processed to preserve the integrity of antigens) are reacted with defined MABs. The binding of the latter is demonstrated by the use of stepwise procedures, whereby a second or subsequent antibody with an attached 'label' is used.

Immunohistological methods, using only a one-stage reaction (direct)—directly labelled MABs—are often too insensitive and too expensive for

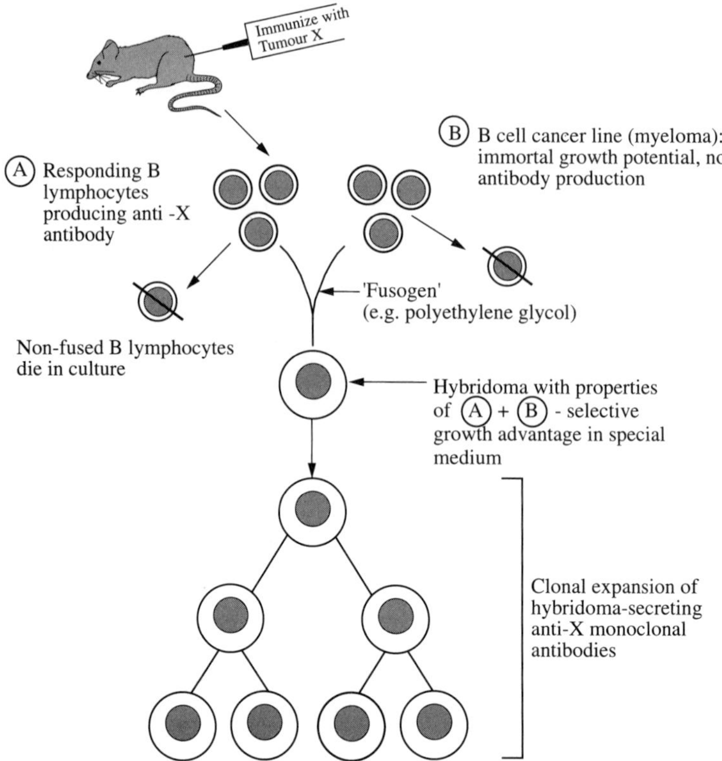

Fig. 9.1. Principle of monoclonal antibody production. The B lymphocytes from the immunized animal produce anti-tumour antibodies. The myeloma cancer cells, when fused with the B cells, confer the genetic information for infinite growth (immortalization). The immunoglobulin secreting B lymphocytes confer on the hybrid the ability to produce antibody. A special tissue culture medium is used which enables the hybridoma to grow and proliferate but results in the death of the unfused B lymphocytes (A) and myeloma cells (B). The secreted monoclonal antibody is harvested from the supernatant.

routine use. The multiple stages in the techniques increases substantially the signal for detection and thus the sensitivity of the technique. The 'labels' used may be enzymes (e.g., peroxidase, alkaline phosphatase) which are exposed to a substrate (usually an organic chemical); the enzyme-substrate reaction results in the deposition of a visible colour product in the vicinity of the tumour antigen-monoclonal antibody reaction complex. Other labels, such as fluorescein are excited by light (UV or laser) and in turn emit light of a wavelength detectable by a UV microscope with appropriate optics or by photodetection systems within machines, such as flow cytometers (see below). Like most laboratory methods, immunohistochemical methods

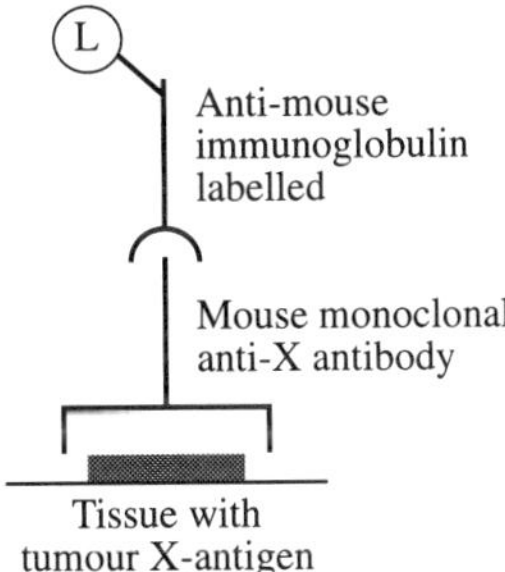

Indirect: 2-stage technique

- Mouse monoclonal with anti-tumour antigen specificity is used as the primary antibody
- The anti-mouse (secondary antibody) can be raised in many species e.g., rabbit, sheep, donkey.
- The label Ⓛ is chemically conjugated to the secondary antibody

Ⓛ, Enzymes: peroxidase, alkaline phosphatase or fluorochromes: fluorescein, rhodamine or Biotin, which binds to complexes of Avidin and Biotin peroxidase (ABC complex)

3-stage technique

- Increases the sensitivity of detection of the bound primary antibody
- Primary and secondary antibodies as in 2 stage technique (see above)
- Tertiary antibody is raised against mouse immunoglobulin and labelledⓁ

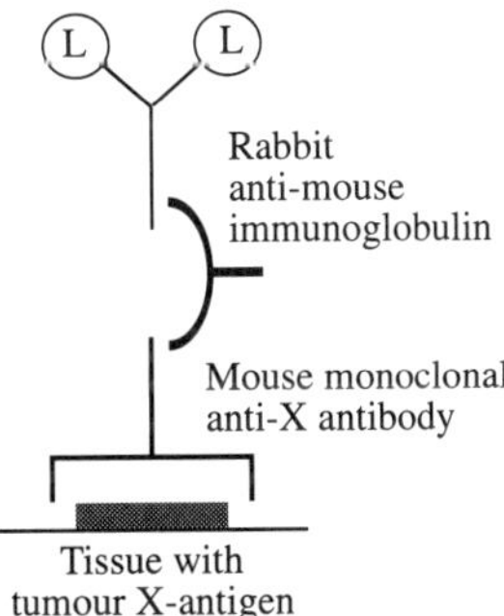

Unlabelled: bridge technique

- The label is bound as an antigen in the tertiary layer immune complex if Ⓛ is peroxidase →PAP system if Ⓛ is alkaline phosphatase → APAAP system
- The linking 'bridge' rabbit anti-mouse immunoglobulin is unlabelled. With some techniques increase in sensitivity can be obtained by using additionally a labelled 'bridge' antibody

Fig. 9.2. Immunohistochemical techniques used in monoclonal antibody detection of tumour antigens/markers. If (L) is a peroxidase enzyme—a chemical substrate (diamino-benzidine) is added and results in deposition of an insoluble brown coloured product. If (L) is a fluorochrome—the tissue is examined in a UV fluourescent microscope. Enzyme (L) labels have advantages over fluorochromes—e.g. tissue reactions visible with a light microscope and a permanent preparation is available.

require attention to methodology, controls (positive and negative), reagent quality assurance, and trained expertise in the interpretation of the immunohistochemical results. Immunohistochemical methods are mainly qualitative or at best are semi-quantitative. (see Polak and Von Noorden 1986)

9.2.3. ELISA and RIA techniques

ELISAs employ many similar methods to the immunohistochemical techniques, but are designed to detect molecules in free solution (Fig. 9.3). In the detection of TAAs in blood and other body fluids, ELISA techniques are based on linking the antibody to the solid phase. If a patient's serum sample contains the antigen, it reacts with the bound antibody. The presence of the antigen is revealed by another reaction with antibody with specificity for that antigen, followed by an enzyme-labelled antiglobulin. The enzyme is reacted with a substrate generating a fluid-phase colour reaction product. The final reaction product can be read manually or more rapidly and efficiently by automated spectrophotometry (ELISA readers). By the incorporation of various standards (e.g., dilutions of antigen and suitable controls) the amounts of tumour antigen in any sample can be accurately quantitated.

Well-known ELISA assays are used to quantitate antigens, such as carcino-embryonic antigen (CEA), CA125, and CA19-9 which are carbohydrate antigens secreted by and associated with various tumours (see below).

RIA

Radioimmunoassays are used in similar situations to ELISA but the indicator systems are based on the emission of various radionuclides linked to antigens or antibodies (e.g., ^{125}I, ^{131}I, ^{3}H). Many laboratories have moved from RIA systems to ELISA, thus avoiding the use of isotopes and their attendant problems. Many ELISA systems are of a sensitivity comparable to the ranges detected by RIA.

9.2.4 Flow cytometry

This is a technique where measurements are made on individual cells as they flow past a sensing device, which is commonly laser light. Many cytometers also have the capability of physically sorting specific cells from a heterogeneous population after they have been analysed. A prerequisite for flow cytometry is optimal tissue (blood and tissue fluids, surgical biopsies, archival histological sections) preparation to obtain a monodispersed population of cells in suspension. Using flow cytometry, multiparametric analysis of single cells can be performed. When the laser light hits the moving cell, the light is dispersed in various directions, which equate to the size of the cell and to its cytosolic properties (e.g., degree of granularity). Also, the nucleic acids within the cell may be labelled with

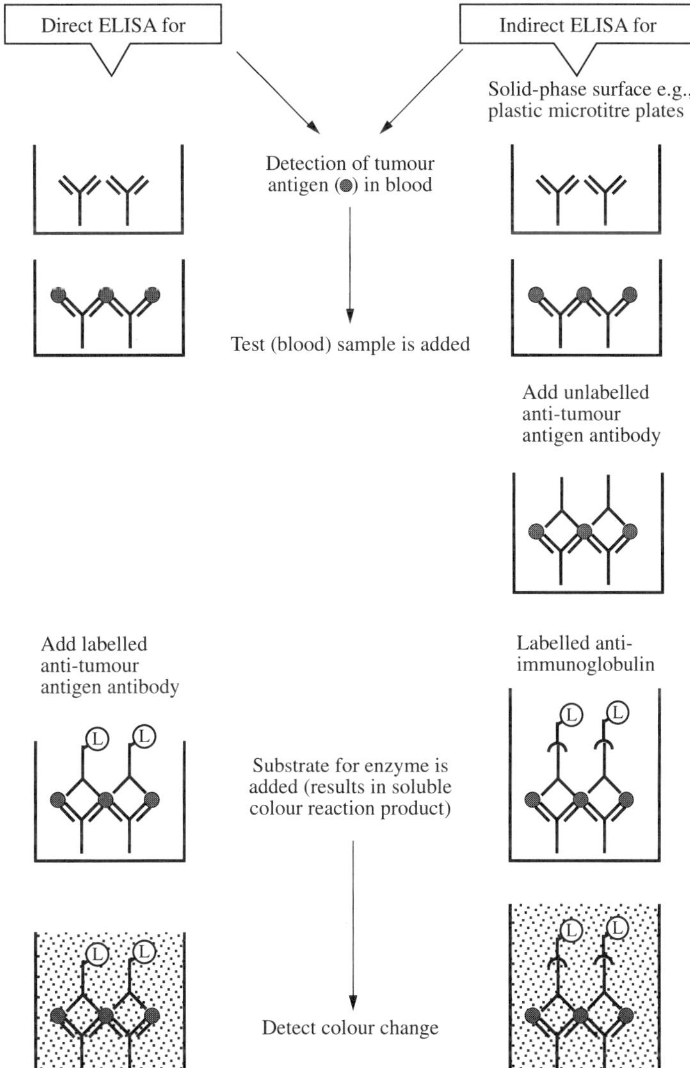

Fig. 9.3. ELISA techniques used to detect and quantitate tumour antigens in fluids. Y—Antibody specific for tumour antigen (●)—bound or adsorbed to solid phase. ●—Tumour antigen/marker-secreted and present in body fluids (blood, synovial etc). L—Enzyme (e.g. peroxidase)—(a) linked to a second tumour antigen (●) specific antibody in the DIRECT ELISA; (b) linked to an anti-immunoglobulin (i.e. anti-anti-tumour immunoglobulin) in the INDIRECT ELISA. This is a more sensitive technique (can detect tumour antigen in nanograms per ml in blood).

certain dyes (e.g., ethidium bromide, propidium iodide) and cell-associated antigens can be reacted with antibodies in immunocytochemical techniques using fluorescent dyes. The various dyes are excited by the laser light and their subsequent light emissions are detected and analysed by the cytometer. Thus information is obtained on the physical parameters of cells, on their DNA/RNA content (and states such as ploidy) and on their antigen expression. These multiparameters provide significant information concerning a cell's phenotype and genotype. Flow cytometry has been used extensively to establish the diagnosis of different leukaemias and lymphomas, and to analyse cytological preparations (washings and aspirates) from carcinomas (e.g., thyroid, cervical, and bladder cancers). Also, documentation of the DNA content of various solid tumours—breast, thyroid, bladder and non-Hodgkin's lymphoma—have been obtained by flow cytometry and correlated with the degree of malignancy on histological evaluation and subsequent prognosis on patient follow-up.

9.2.5 Tumour marker assays in laboratory practice

Defining the tissue origin of anaplastic tumours

Markedly dedifferentiated (anaplastic) tumours may prove difficult to characterize precisely and to define accurately their tissue of origin, using classic histological methods. A simple panel of MABs has proved extremely valuable in this situation. The antibodies used are directed to intermediate filaments, which are proteins which constitute a major part of the cell cytoskeleton. Different cell types, even when malignant, maintain their characteristic intermediate filaments. Thus, normal epithelial cells and their corresponding tumours (carcinomas), possess the intermediate filament *cytokeratin*, whilst muscle cells contain *desmin*, mesenchymal cells *vimentin*, and neural cells *neurofilaments*. Table 9.1 summarizes the pattern of activity

Table 9.1. Monoclonal antibody specificities and immunohistochemical reactivity

Anaplastic Tumour type	**IF[a] cytokeratin**	**IF desmin**	**IF vimentin**	**LCA[b]**	**IF neurofilament**
Carcinoma	+	–	–(+)	–	–
Lymphoma	–	–	+(–)	+	–
Melanoma	–	–	+	–	–
Neural tumours	–	–	–	–	+
Rhabdomyosarcoma	–	+	+	–	–
Leiomyosarcoma	–	+	–	–	–
Ewing	–	–	+	–	–

[a] IF, Intermediate filament; [b] LCA, leucocyte common antigen (CD45) is not an (IF), it is a macromolecular protein restricted to leucocytes.

found using a panel of MABs to intermediate filaments in the diagnosis of anaplastic cancers. Table 9.2 illustrates some tumour markers and appropriate assays used in clinical laboratory practice. Plate 1 illustrates immunocytochemical staining reactions (of several tumours for the relevant TAA) used in clinical diagnosis/management of cancer patients.

9.3 Assessment of lymphocytes

Qualitative, quantitative, and functional assays of lymphocytes *in vitro* and *in vivo* provide an opportunity to characterize an individual's state of immune responsiveness. The assays include: (1) *in vitro* counts of total T, B, and T subsets of lymphocytes; (2) *in vitro* functional assays of T and B cell responses to antigens and mitogens; (3) *in vivo* functional tests of T cells (CMI) as manifested by DTH reactions in skin tests; (4) *in vitro* assays of functional cytotoxicity tests for NK and LAK cell activity.

9.3.1 Quantification of lymphocytes

Counts of total T, B, and T subset lymphocyte populations

Quantification of the lymphoid populations are useful: (1) in the monitoring of HIV infection (see Chapter 8, Fig. 8.3); (2) in the investigation of other immune deficiency states suspected from a clinical history of persistent, recurrent, serious or unusual infections; (3) in the determination of the type of cells involved in a probable lympho-proliferative malignancy; and (4) to determine whether a persistent blood lymphocytosis is benign or malignant, e.g., normal B cells in blood have approximately 50 per cent positive kappa- and 50 per cent positive lambda-bearing cells. In contrast, malignant B cell proliferations are monoclonal and usually only one light chain is detected.

Quantification is performed using samples of fresh anticoagulated blood or partially purified mononuclear cell populations obtained by density gradient sedimentation. The blood is diluted with phosphate buffered saline and layered over a suitable dense separation substance such as Ficoll-Isopaque (SG: 1.077) and centrifuged (450 *g* for 30 min). Blood cells move differentially through such a separation medium, and mononuclear cells comprising mainly lymphocytes (with some monocytes) collect at the interface of the gradient and the upper plasma layer; red blood cells and granulocytes form a pellet at the bottom of the centrifuge tube. Whole blood or partially purified cells are incubated with MABs to various T and B cell-associated CD antigens (e.g., CD3, CD4, CD8, CD19; see Chapter 1) and to more specific markers, e.g., antigen-specific T and B cell receptors (TCR and SmIg) on the lymphocytes. The binding of the MABs are revealed by incubation with anti-mouse antibody reagents which are labelled with

Table 9.2. Tumour-associated markers and immunological assays

Tumour-associated marker/antigen	Tumour	Assay	Comment
1. Intermediate filaments (IF)	See Table 9.1	Immunohistology	Additional antibodies may contribute to further characterization of anaplastic tumours.
2. Carcino-embryonic antigen (CEA)	Colonic and other gastrointestinal tumours	Tissue: immunohistology Serum: ELISA/RIA	Pre- and post-surgery monitoring of serum CEA in patients with known colonic cancer.
3. Carbohydrate-associated antigens: CA19–9	Gastrointestinal tumours	Tissue: immunohistology Serum: ELISA/RIA	Not specific for a particular cancer. Serum assays—shows some selectivity in detecting pancreatic cancer.
CA125	Ovarian cancer-associated	Tissue: immunohistology Serum: ELISA/RIA	Serum ELISA for CA125-good for monitoring ovarian cancer patients. Tissue does not react with mucinous ovarian tumours, found in other carcinomas.
CA15–3	Breast cancer	Tissue: immunohistology Serum: ELISA/RIA	Not specific for breast cancer.
4. Placental alkaline phosphatase	Seminoma and some carcinomas	Tissue: immunohistology Serum: ELISA/RIA	Good marker for seminoma metastases. - Positive in some ovarian cancers. - ELISA/RIA used to monitor seminoma patients. Antibody also useful in radionuclide 'imaging' techniques *in vivo*.

5. p97 – melanoma-associated antigen	Malignant melanoma	Tissue:	immunohistology	Positive in pigmented and amelanotic melanoma. Useful in defining metastases with occult primary.
6. Glial fibrillary acid protein (GFAP)	Brain tumours	Tissue:	immunohistology	Useful in distinguishing glial tumours from metastases in the brain from non-central nervous system sites.
7. Alpha-fetoprotein	Hepatoma Malignant testicular tumours	Tissue: Serum:	immunohistology ELISA/RIA	Very useful for serum monitoring of patients with tumours, and following therapy.
8. Human chorionic gonadotrophin	Trophoblastic tumours, gestational chorio-carcinoma, testicular and ovarian tumours	Tissue: Serum:	immunohistology ELISA/RIA	Serology – used pre- and post-surgery and for patient monitoring.
9. Thyroglobulin	Thyroid tumours (papillary, follicular, and anaplastic)	Tissue: Serum:	immunohistology ELISA/RIA	Pre- and post-surgery serology.
10. Prostate specific antigen	Prostatic cancer	Tissue: Serum:	immunohistology ELISA/RIA	Local tissue invasion – differentiates bladder from prostate cancer. Serology ELISA – antigen increased in metastatic disease.

Table 9.2. cont'd

Tumour-associated marker/antigen	Tumour	Assay	Comment
11. Oestrogen receptor protein	Breast cancer (Ovarian cancer)	Tissue: immunohistology RIA: ligand-binding tissue homogenate assay	Prognostic; influences therapy decisions.
12. CD antigens (Panels of monoclonals; see Chapter 1)	T/B cell lineage and null leukaemias and lymphomas	Tissue: immunohistology Cells in suspension: Flow cytometry	Diagnosis—subtyping: prognostic monitoring of cells for remission, relapse status.
13. Kappa and lambda staining	B cell tumours	Tissue: immunohistology Cells in suspension: Flow cytometry	Defining monoclonality (neoplastic nature) of B cell populations.
14. Immunoglobulins, monoclonal proteins	Multiple myeloma, other plasma cell dyscracias	Tissue: smears Biopsies: immunohistology Serum: electrophoresis Cells: flow cytometry	Staining for kappa and lambda light chains often reveal the monoclonal (neoplastic) nature of B lineage proliferations.
15. Ectopic hormones (e.g., ACTH, ADH)	Lung tumours Oat cell carcinoma	Tissue: immunohistology Serum: ELISA/RIA	Can be used to evaluate response to therapy.

enzymes (see Fig. 9.2) or fluorescent probes. The labelled cells are quantified manually under direct vision (microscopy) or by automation, e.g., flow cytometry (see above) and expressed as percentages and absolute counts relative to the total lymphocyte count and established normal ranges.

9.3.2 *In vitro* functional assays

T and B lymphocyte activation following reaction to antigens (soluble or cell-associated) or mitogens (see Chapter 1) results in many biochemical and cellular events involving cell synthesis of DNA/RNA, secretion of lymphokines, and expression of activation markers, such as the interleukin-2 (IL-2) receptor and cell mitosis. *In vitro* functional assays of T lymphocytes are useful: (1) in the investigation of possible CMI deficiency including HIV infection; (2) as part of the documentation of a potential recipient's reactivity to donor cell-associated antigens which may result in acute allograft rejection. The *in vitro* mixed lymphocyte reaction (MLR) (also called mixed lymphocyte culture (MLC)) and cell-mediated lympholysis (CML) assays are useful correlates of *in vivo* events in transplantation rejection (see Chapter 2).

Figure 9.4 indicates T cell recognition, activation, and some subsequent events which follow antigen recognition. The numbered events (1–5) can be assayed as follows:

1. DNA/RNA synthesis can be measured by incorporation of radiolabelled nucleotide precursors in the cultures of responding lymphocytes and stimulatory cells. The antigen-bearing stimulatory cells are rendered non-responsive prior to mixing with the lymphocytes by irradiation or by

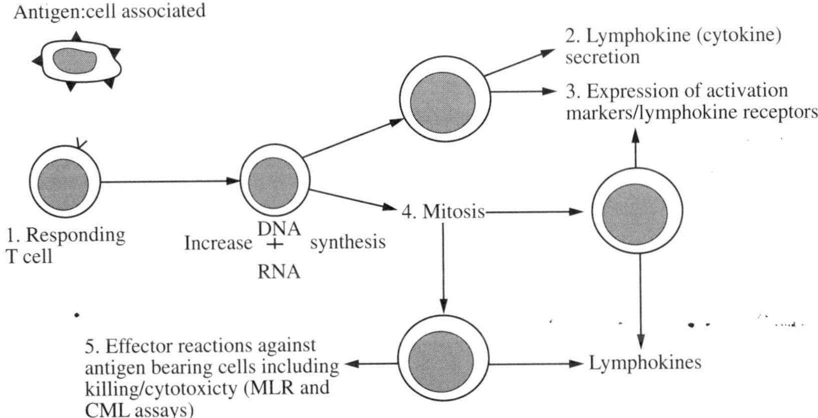

Fig. 9.4 Measurable consequences of T cell reaction to 'non-self' antigens on a cell.

chemicals (mitomycin C). If the lymphocytes respond to the stimulatory cells they will undergo blast transformation and cell division and incorporate the radiolabelled nucleotide precursors (e.g., tritiated thymidine) into their newly synthesized DNA, which is detected by measuring the disintegrations emitted per unit time in a beta counter.

2. The responding T lymphocytes may secrete such lymphokines as IL-2 or IFN-γ which can be measured in ELISA, RIA, or by bioassays in which known *in vitro* cell lines (Jurkat) respond to the addition of lymphokine, by growth and proliferation.

3. Responding T cells can be documented by their expression of activation markers – IL-2 receptor (CD25) or HLA-DR molecules. These can be quantitated by direct or indirect immunocytochemical methods, manually or by flow cytometry.

4. The mitotic events of the responding T cells can be documented by counting the exponential increase in cells, or by radioactive tracing of incorporated isotopically labelled DNA precursor molecules. These approaches are commonly employed in the MLR test, where inactivated (irradiated, pre-treated with mitomycin C) donor blood lymphocytes are incubated with normal recipient blood lymphocytes. If the recipient's cells possess significant anti-donor cell reactivity it is demonstrated by increased cell uptake of tritiated (^{3}H) thymidine and/or increased cell mitosis. Such a positive MLR would tend to indicate a heightened probability of graft rejection *in vivo*. A variant of this assay is the mixed lymphocyte tumour cell reaction (MLTR), where the stimulatory cells are autologous or allogeneic tumour cells (isolated from tumours, cell lines).

5. A further assay (CML) documents the killing of viable donor-stimulatory cells (labelled with chromium 51 (^{51}Cr)), following incubation (4 to 24 hours) with recipient's lymphocytes (activated T killer cells). MLR and CML are used to estimate pre-sensitization and histocompatibility in clinical transplantation (see Chapter 2). Cellular assays are time consuming and require careful setting up with appropriate controls. Assays are usually set up in triplicates and each reaction uses the lowest number of cells, e.g., 5×10^4 cells per well or tube in 0.2 to 0.5 ml of tissue culture medium.

9.3.3 *In vivo* assays of CMI—DTH skin test

Injection of standard 'recall' antigens (i.e. antigens to which an individual has been exposed to in the past and, therefore, possesses the appropriate memory T cells) into the dermal layers of the skin, results in activation of the specific memory T cells, secretion of lymphokines, and attraction of other T lymphocytes and macrophages-monocytes into the skin site resulting in a classical DTH skin lesion – redness, oedema, swelling, etc., some 48 to 72 hours following antigen injection. This test gives an overall analysis of an individuals T cell immune competence, i.e., from the earliest T cell receptor-antigen recognition to the generation of the effector cells and reactions. Commercial preparations of sterile 'recall' antigens, at standard doses, are employed—derived from microbial extracts, mumps virus, antigens of streptococci (streptokinase/streptodornase), and antigens of fungi (*Candida, Trichophyton*). The antigens and controls are injected intradermally (e.g., 0.1 ml of a defined preparation into the injection sites) or applied using multiple small puncture needles and are read at 48–72 hours to document the extent of the characteristic erythematous-indurated lesion.

9.3.4 NK and LAK cell assays

In vitro, the possible anti-tumour cell killing abilities of these mononuclear cells (Chapter 1, Section 1.5.3) can be documented by cytotoxicity assays, using well-defined target cell lines. Human NK cell activity is demonstrated using the target cell line *K562*. LAK cell killing is monitored using the *Daudi* cell line, which is resistant to NK activity. When LAK activity is evident, then killing of both K562 and of Daudi is clearly demonstrable.

The target cells which are in suspension, are labelled with ^{51}Cr and incubated with the test effector mononuclear cells at defined target to effector cell ratios. Centrifugation prior to incubation at 37 °C for 4 hours ensures intimate contact and subsequent interaction following the incubation; culture supernatants are collected and isotope emission (^{51}Cr) is measured in a gamma counter. The ^{51}Cr, which labels the cytosol proteins in the living cells is released into the supernatant following cell membrane damage and osmotic lysis of target cells. Thus, counts of radioactivity in the supernatant and the target cells, relative to various controls, give a measure of the effector cell cytotoxicity. *In vitro* LAK activity can be generated by incubating NK cells, or mononuclear cell preparations, with IL-2 for 2 to 3 days. Certain MABs CD16 and CD56, are used in immunocytochemical assays to phenotypically define and quantitate NK and LAK cells.

9.4 Tissue typing

Much of the rapid progress in organ transplantation which has been achieved in the past 25 years, is due to the increased understanding and control of the major impediment to successful transplantation—immunological rejection. The success rate of organ transplantation in humans is greatly enhanced by matching of the major histocompatibility antigens (or human leucocyte antigens—HLA antigens) which are present in all tissues and on blood lymphocytes. This latter fact is fortuitous, because tissue typing (or the determination of major histocompatibility antigens) can be conveniently carried out using blood lymphocytes. The human major histocompatibility gene locus, found on the short arm of chromosome 6, is a complex and highly polymorphic region coding for class I and class II antigens (major histocompatibility complex—MHC antigens) as well as some complement components (see Chapters 1 and 2). The class I antigens A (23 allelic types), B (49), and C (about 10) are *typed* using freshly isolated and viable blood lymphocytes in an antibody-based, complement-dependent cytotoxicity test (Fig. 9.5). Whilst MHC class II or D-related (DR) antigens (present on B cells, monocytes, dendritic cells, and activated T lymphocytes) were originally detected by time-consuming (5 day) MLRs requiring standard typing (stimulator) cells, these may now also be identified serologically on B lymphocytes of prospective graft recipients in a similar fashion to that for detection of HLA-A, B, and C antigens. MLR assays are nevertheless still performed in the situation of bone marrow transplantation, along with serological assays.

In principle, the cells to be typed are added to the wells of a microtitre ('Terasaki') plate containing monospecific anti-HLA anti-sera, obtained from multiparous women or from patients who have received multiple blood transfusions. If antibodies are bound, complement (source: normal rabbit serum) is fixed and the cells are lysed. The dead cells are identified by an indicator dye (trypan blue), which renders the cells readily identifiable under the microscope. If most (> 90 per cent) of the lymphocytes are killed by a given anti-serum, then they are presumed to have expressed the relevant HLA antigen recognized by the typing antibody. The duration of the test is approximately 2 hours for HLA-class I antigens and approximately 4 hours for HLA-DR typing, the additional time being required for preparation of B lymphocytes. Tissue typing is a complex and expensive technique which is only available in specialized centres usually in conjunction with an organ transplantation programme.

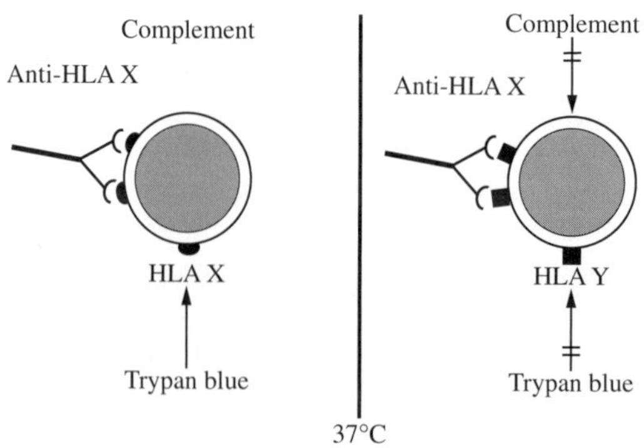

Fig. 9.5. Microcytotoxicity test for HLA antigens; lysis HLAX cells.

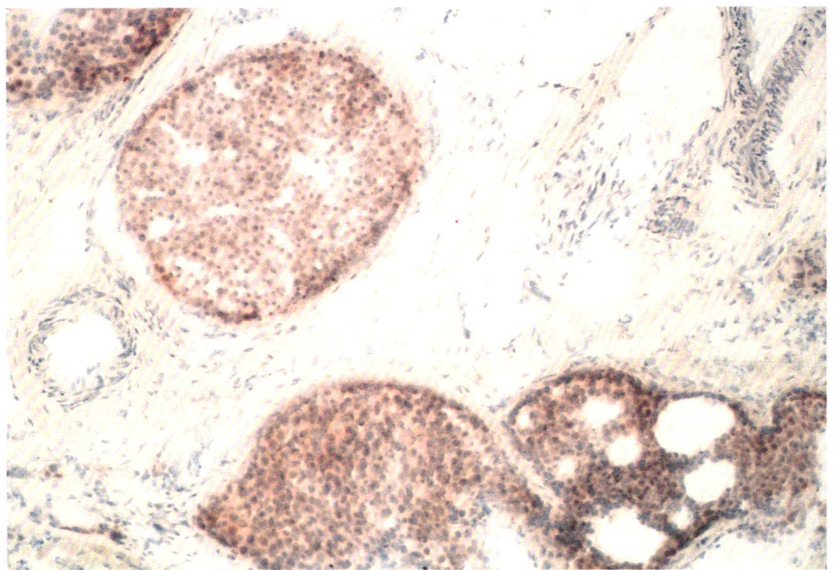

Plate 1 (a) Positive staining (red) of oestrogen receptor protein (ORP) in an intraduct breast carcinoma using a monoclonal antibody to ORP. (APAAP method with blue haematoxylin counterstain.)

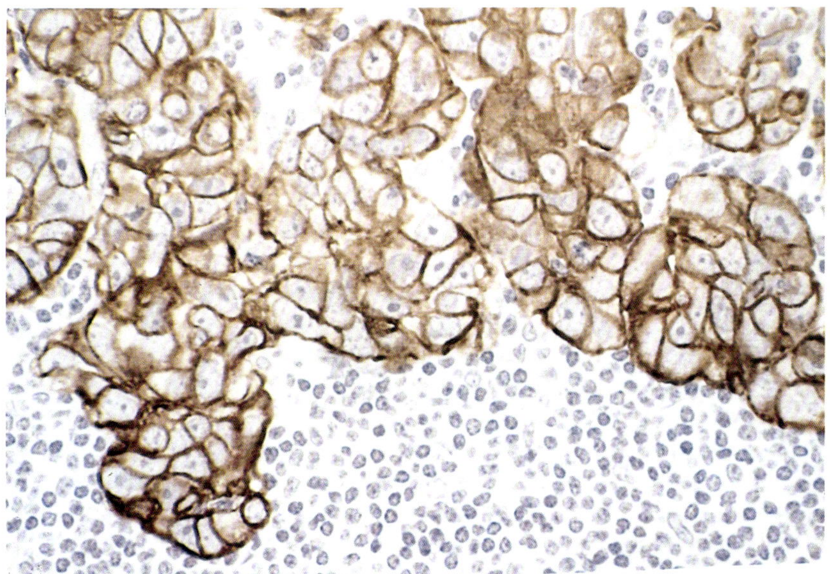

Plate 1 (b) Positive staining (brown) of metastatic deposits of anaplastic carcinoma cells in a lymph node using a monoclonal antibody to cytokeratin. The adjacent lymphoid tissue with the blue haematoxylin nuclear counterstain is negative. (PAP method.)

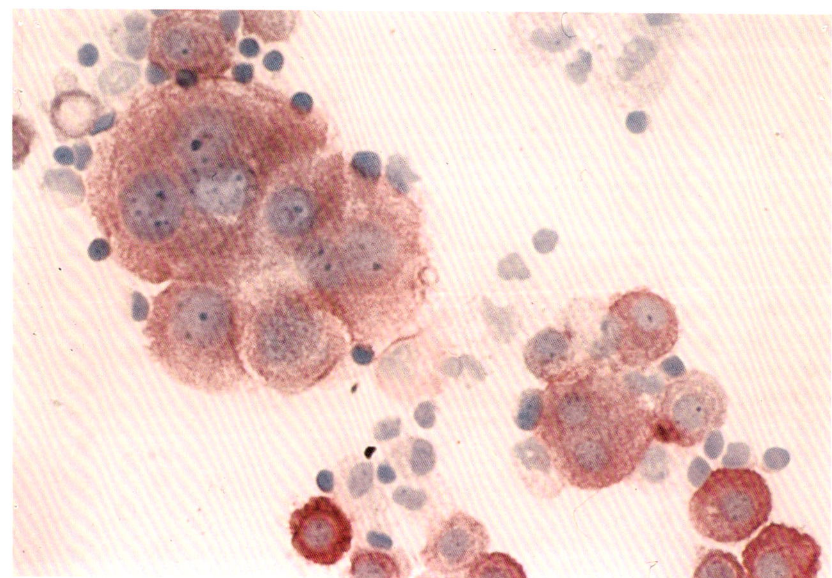

Plate 1 (c) Positive staining (red) of clusters of ovarian cancer cells obtained from an ascitic fluid. Cytospin preparations were reacted with a monoclonal antibody to the CA125 antigen. Smaller individual normal mesothelial cells are also positive. (APAAP method.)

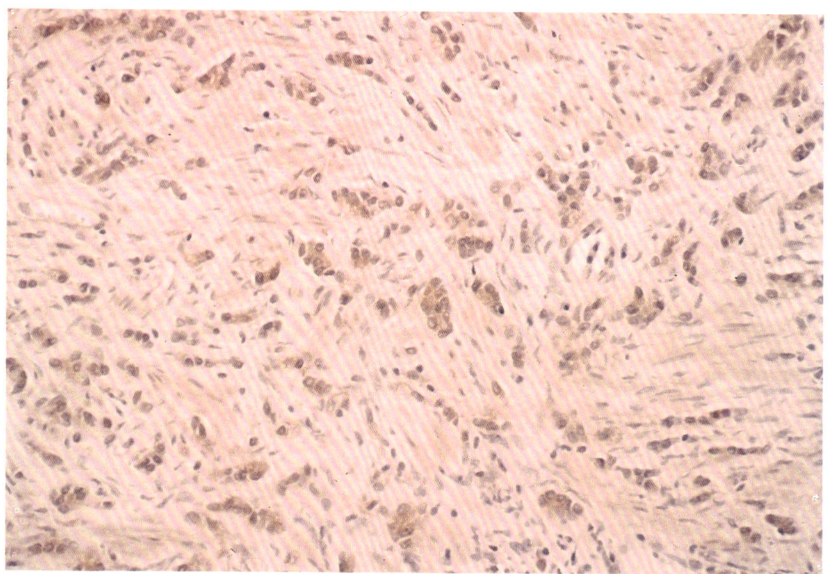

Plate 1 (d) Positive staining (brown) of infiltrating nests of anaplastic prostatic carcinoma cells, using a monoclonal antibody to prostate specific antigen. (ABC method.)

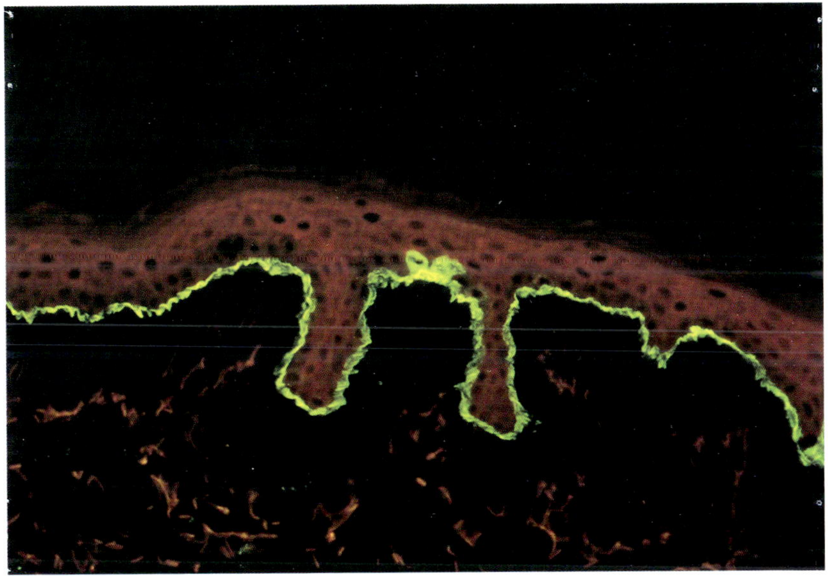

Plate 2 (a) Direct immunofluorescence (IF) showing positive staining (green) of the epidermal–dermal junction of *in vivo* bound IgG anti-epidermal basement membrane antibodies in a skin biopsy from a patient with bullous pemphigoid. Staining was also positive with anti-complement component antibody. (Direct IF using cryostat sections of skin biopsy.)

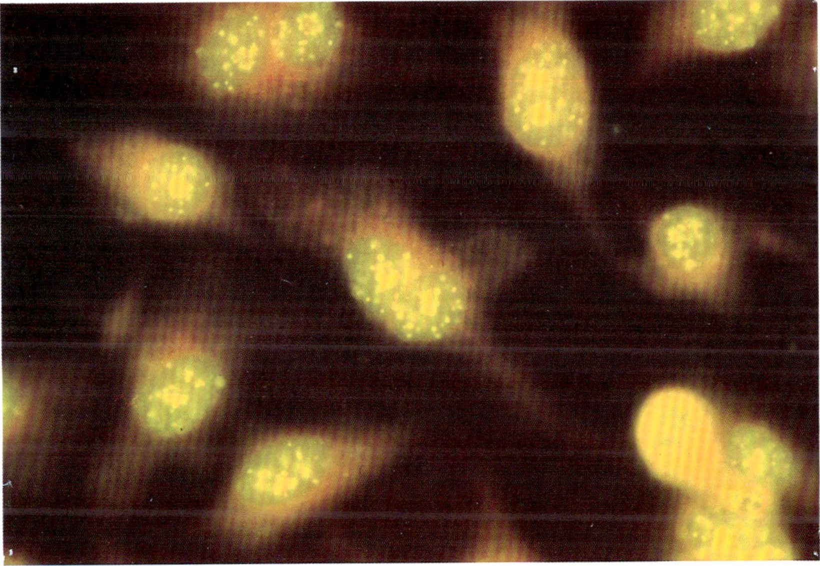

Plate 2 (b) Positive staining for Anti-Centromere antibody (note dot positivity of the centromeres in the metaphase nuclei) in a patient with idiopathic Raynaud's disease. (Indirect IF substrate–carcinoma cell line HEP-2.)

(c)

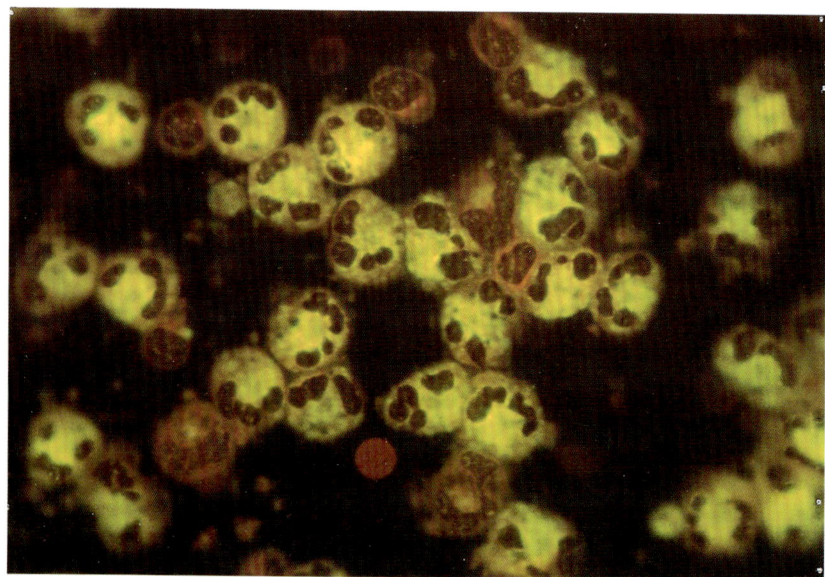

(d)

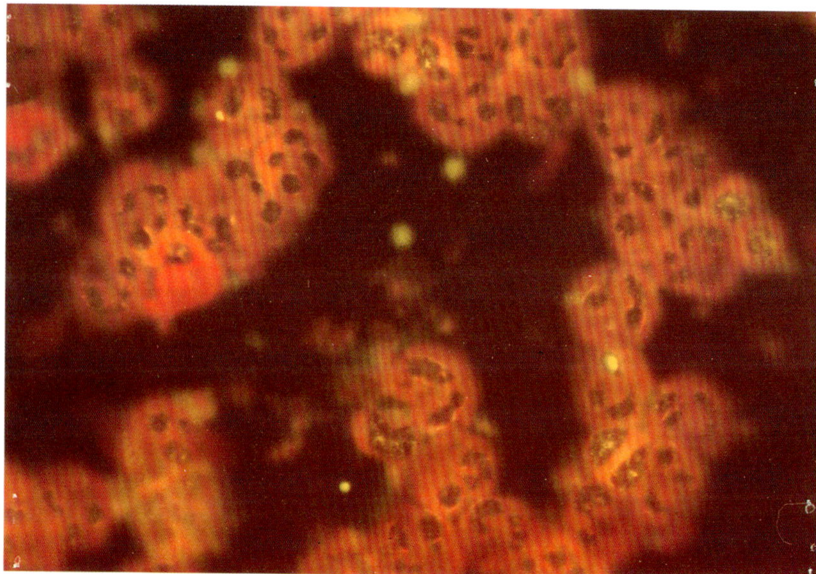

Plate 2 (c) (d) Detection of Antibody to Neutrophil Cytoplasmic Antigen (ANCA). A 25-year old patient presents to ENT surgeons with signs and symptoms of inflammatory lesions involving the maxillary sinus and oro-pharynx; a diagnosis of early Wegener's granulomatosis was suspected. The indirect immunofluorescence test for ANCA was positive with the patient's serum (c) and negative with control serum (d). (Indirect IF passage using cytospin preparations of human neutrophils.)

9.4.1 Future methods of HLA typing

It is now possible to apply molecular biological techniques (see Section 9.9) to human tissue typing and there is every indication that, in the future, these methods which have numerous applications, may supercede immunological procedures. Thus, HLA-class I and II specific DNA probes, which detect restriction fragment length polymorphisms (RFLPs) are currently under evaluation. In addition, such gene probes have the potential to distinguish between defective antigen expression and gene deletion.

9.5 Assessment of neutrophils and monocytes

9.5.1 Assays of phagocytic cell function

Phagocytic cells (neutrophil polymorphs and mononuclear phagocytes) play crucial roles in the engulfment and killing of bacteria and fungi and in the removal of damaged tissue within the body (See Chapter 1, Section 1.5.2). In order to exercise these functions, however, they must be able to locate, recognize, ingest, and subsequently destroy/digest the offending material via the action of lysosomal enzymes. Primary deficiencies of such phagocytic cell functions are rare. Included in this category is chronic granulomatous disease, in which there is defective intracellular killing of (otherwise normally) engulfed bacteria or fungi due to failure of the cells to produce reactive oxygen intermediates. Other rare causes are Chediak–Higashi syndrome, in which lysosomal abnormalities predispose to pyogenic infections which can prove fatal, and the lazy leucocyte syndrome, characterized by defective neutrophil chemotactic responses. More common are secondary defects in phagocyte function, which may result from infection, malnutrition, burns or trauma (Chapters 4–6). It should also be noted that deficient phagocyte function *in vivo* may be a consequence of defective production/inadequate levels of opsonins, i.e., molecules which bind to particles to be phagocytosed and to receptors on phagocytic cells, thereby acting as a bridge between the two (e.g., IgG, C3b, and C-reactive protein).

Absolute numbers of circulating neutrophils and monocytes are readily determined from total and differential white blood cell counts. As with tests of T cell-mediated immunity, assays of phagocytic cell function, in general, are difficult to perform and labour-intensive. In common with the former assays, they should only be performed if the clinical features indicate immune deficiency. Neutrophils are separated from anticoagulated whole blood by centrifuging on Ficoll-Hypaque; they are obtained from the centrifuged pellet (red cells plus granulocytes) after hypo-osmotic lysis of the erythrocytes and removal of the red cell ghosts. Monocytes, on the other hand, are separated from lymphocytes, both isolated at the

Ficoll–plasma interface, by their capacity to adhere to glass or plastic surfaces from which the latter can be subsequently removed.

9.5.2 Assays of chemotaxis

The capacity of a patient's neutrophils or monocytes to respond to standard chemotactic stimuli (e.g., casein, or the synthetic peptide f-met-leu-phe) can be determined by placing the cells suspended in medium on one side of a chamber ('Boyden' chamber) separated by a thin membrane (either polycarbonate or nitrocellulose membranes may be used) from medium containing the chemotactic stimulus (Fig. 9.6). After incubation at 37°C for 1 to 3 hours, the membrane is stained and examined microscopically, for the extent of cell migration (distance migrated or number of cells reaching lower surface) towards the chemo-attractant. Incorporation of normal control standards is essential in all these cellular assays.

9.5.3 Opsonization and phagocytosis

Defects in the phagocytic ability of patients' cells, or in the capacity of patients' sera to facilitate the opsonization of particles via complement, can be examined in 'cross-over' studies in which the cells are incubated with particles, such as yeast cells (which activate the alternative complement pathway directly). Suitable phagocytic particles include latex beads, or red blood cells coated with immunoglobulin with or without complement components, yeasts or bacteria. Following incubation and ingestion the cells are usually fixed and stained to optimize counting.

9.5.4 Bacterial killing

Standard assays of intracellular killing (e.g., *Staphylococcus aureus*) involve incubation of the cells with live organisms followed by removal of non-ingested bacteria by centrifugation, then release (by osmotic lysis of the phagocytes) and subsequent culture of viable organisms. The number of viable organisms is related inversely to the extent of intracellular killing.

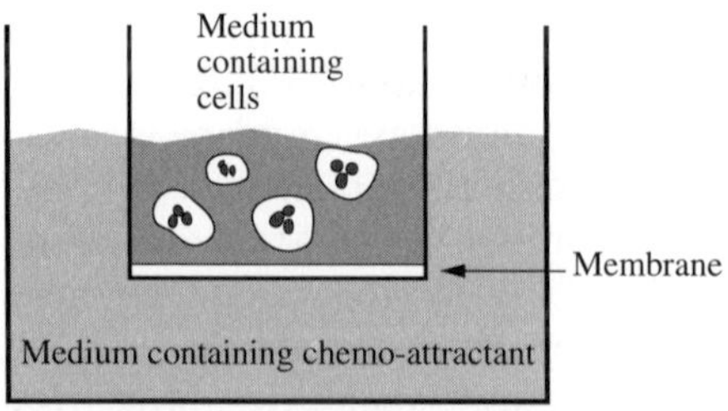

Fig. 9.6. Schematic diagram of chamber used for testing neutrophil or monocyte chemoattractant ability.

9.5.5 Quantification of the respiratory burst (metabolic function)

Particle ingestion by phagocytic cells induces a respiratory burst which can be quantified by the intracellular reduction of yellow nitroblue tetrazolium (NBT) dye to insoluble blue crystals which can be counted under the light microscope or extracted and quantified spectrophotometrically. A widely available screening test which assesses total function is the 'activated NBT test', in which the phagocytes are first primed with a standard amount of bacterial endotoxin.

9.6 Detection of autoantibodies

Testing for autoantibodies (see Chapter 8) is usually performed using the following assays:

1 *Immunofluorescence techniques*

(a) *Direct*. In this method fluorescein-conjugated anti-sera (anti-human immunoglobulin and complement) are added directly to surgical biopsy specimens (e.g., skin and renal biopsies), to demonstrate *in vivo* bound autoantibodies and activated/deposited complement components. Such assays are used in the differential diagnosis of skin lesions, associated with bullous disorders and putative connective issue diseases (e.g., SLE). They also play a significant role in the diagnosis of renal pathology (see Plate 2(a)).

(b) *Indirect*. This method employs substrates (tissues) of animal or human origin which contain the relevant autoantigens. Patients' sera (primary layer in Fig. 9.2) are incubated with the substrate and any circulating autoantibodies bind to their respective tissue autoantigens. Following repeated washings, to remove unreacted serum proteins, the presence of bound autoantibodies is revealed by a secondary layer (Fig. 9.2) consisting of serum containing fluorescein-labelled anti-human immunoglobulin. Controls (positive and negative) are included in the assays and the distribution of the staining patterns, in relation to tissue cell type and anatomic locations, is determined. For indirect methods many autoantigens, especially those associated with non-organ specific autoimmunity, e.g., nucleic acids, smooth muscle, and mitochondrial antigens, are not species specific, hence substrates, such as rat and mouse tissues, can be used. Substrates (commonly fresh material) are snap frozen in liquid nitrogen, and sectioned on cryostats thus resulting in optimal antigen preservation. Other autoantigens (Chapter 8) especially for organ specific autoantibodies are much more species specific, thus human surgical or early post-mortem tissue or closely related primate substrates have to be used.

2. Haemagglutination assays

Haemagglutination assays using red blood cells (of various species coated with autoantigens) as indicator particles, are used to detect various autoantibodies, e.g., anti-thyroglobulin and microsomal antibodies in autoimmune thyroid diseases—the antigens are chemically cross-linked to the red cell membrane. Incubation with several dilutions of the patient's serum are performed; if autoantibodies are present they induce agglutination (clumping) of the red cells which can be readily seen in a microtitre plate. In some assays, such as the Rose–Waaler, for detecting classical IgM rheumatoid factor, the red cells, to which are bound sub-agglutinating doses of IgG anti-red cell antibodies, are used as antigen. The rheumatoid factor in a patient's serum then interacts mainly with the Fc region of the IgG resulting in agglutination of the red cells. *In vivo* generated pathological anti-erythrocyte antibodies, as are found in autoimmune haemolytic anaemias, are demonstrated by the classic direct and indirect Coombs tests.

The end-point of haemagglutination assays can be quantitated and expressed as a titre, i.e., degree of red cell agglutination, or be expressed with respect to national or international standards as international units. Laboratories will quote a range of values for interpreting such autoantibody assays.

3. Other assays

ELISA systems are being used more in the detection of autoantibodies, e.g., double-stranded-native DNA for diagnosis of SLE, or thyroglobulin for thyroid autoimmunity. The antigens are linked to plastic solid phases and patients' sera at various dilutions, are then added. If autoantibodies are present they bind to the fixed antigen and their presence is revealed by labelled anti-immunoglobulin reagents. *RIAs* (see above) are used in the detection of anti-cardiolipin and other anti-phospholipid antibodies which are found in subgroups of SLE patients and those prone to episodes of recurrent thrombosis. The latter may present to general or vascular surgeons, or to obstetricians with recurrent abortions. Plate 2 illustrates some examples of autoantibody assays used in clinical practice.

9.7 Investigations of immunoglobulins-antibodies

9.7.1. Qualitative and quantitative immunoglobulin assays

The detection, analysis, and measurement of immunoglobulins present in plasma or other body fluids depends on their physico-chemical and immunochemical properties as proteins. Immunoglobulin (Ig) abnormalities *per se* or more commonly, other pathological conditions affecting the cells (plasma cells) which produce immunoglobulins, occur in a variety of conditions including immunodeficiency states, infection, lymphoproliferative disorders, liver disease, autoimmune disorders, and chronic inflammation. Detectable abnormalities of Igs include the following:

1. Absolute increase/decrease in the concentration of one of the five immunoglobulin classes.
2. Excessive production of a homogeneous (monoclonal) immunoglobulin (which may indicate multiple myeloma).
3. Excessive production of free immunoglobulin light chains (kappa, lambda or both).
4. Increased production of polymeric immunoglobulins.
5. Production of 'cryoglobulins' – immunoglobulins or other serum proteins which come out of solution at temperatures below 37°C.

Qualitative investigations

Serum. The initial screening test of fresh sera for possible immunoglobulin abnormalities is *serum protein electrophoresis*, which is usually conducted using a cellulose acetate membrane ('strip') as the support medium. A normal serum sample is always run under the same conditions. Following the deposition of samples at the cathodal end of the membrane and the application of an electric current for 45 minute, the membrane is removed from the electrophoresis tank and the protein bands visualized using an appropriate dye, e.g., Coomassie blue or nigrosin. Normal serum separates into pre-albumin, albumin, and five globulin bands, the most cathodal of which is the broad γ-globulin band formed by the immunoglobulins. The principal value of this screening test is in the detection of excessive production of homogeneous immunoglobulin, which is visualized by discrete bands (M-bands), usually in the γ-globulin region. Whenever an M-band is detected or suspected, the serum is subjected to *immuno-electrophoresis* to ascertain the monoclonal nature of the Ig. The principle of this test is similar to serum protein electrophoresis,. however, agar gel is used as the support medium and serum is placed in wells punched in the agar. Following electrophoretic separation of the proteins, troughs are carefully cut between the wells, parallel to the axis of migration, and filled with anti-sera specific to the Ig classes or light chain (κ or λ) isotypes. Proteins reacting with these anti-sera are precipitated (after 12–24 hours) within the agar and subsequently stained; non-precipitated proteins are removed by washing.

An alternative approach to the typing of monoclonal immunoglobulins, which has the advantage of speed and sensitivity, is *immunofixation*. In this assay, membranes pre-soaked in specific anti-sera are overlaid onto the electrophoresed sample (cellulose acetate or agar gel) with protein precipitation (immunofixation) occurring within 2 hours. Whenever serum cryoglobulins are suspected, blood sampling, clotting, and serum separation must take place at 37°C. Thereafter, the serum is maintained at 4°C for 24–48 hours, after which any resulting precipitate is centrifuged and washed at 4°C. Re-dissolving of the precipitate (at 37°C) is followed by immunoelectrophoresis or immunofixation. Cryoglobulins may be monoclonal (myeloma) or mixed, macroglobulin proteins (usually IgM–IgG complexes) associated in the latter instance with chronic inflammatory autoimmune disease.

Urine. Minute free quantities of immunoglobulin light chains are present in the urine of all normal individuals. Whilst abnormal levels of heterogeneous, free, light chains are encountered in conditions associated with increased Ig production, free monoclonal light chains (Bence–Jones proteins) are encountered in cases of myelomatosis. Routine investigation of suspected Bence–Jones proteins first requires concentration of the urine (e.g., by ultrafiltration), followed by cellulose acetate electrophoresis and then immunoelectrophoresis or immunofixation to confirm the presence of either monoclonal κ or λ free light chains. Analysis of urine is deemed essential in myeloma and in any other condition in which an M-band has been detected.

Quantitative analysis

Measurements of serum immunoglobulins are essential in cases of suspected immune deficiency, in patients with severe or repeated infections, and in lympho-proliferative disease. They may also prove helpful in the diagnosis of a variety of other conditions, including liver disease and autoimmune disorders. Each laboratory establishes its own normal population ranges, according to in-house methods and standards. The basis of the most convenient and commonly used assay (single radial immunodiffusion) is immunoprecipitation, i.e., the formation of precipitates when antigen (immunoglobulin) and appropriate precipitating antibody are present in optimal proportions.

Single radial immunodiffusion (SRID)

In this assay, precipitating (usually polyclonal) antibody directed specifically against the heavy chain of the immunoglobulin class to be measured, is mixed with molten agar and the resulting mixture poured onto a glass or plastic plate. After setting, a series of holes is punched in the agar to which samples of test or control serum (or other body fluids) are added. Commercial plates, based on this principle for the measurement of either immunoglobulins or certain complement components (e.g., C3, C4), are readily available.

As the antigen (immunoglobulin) diffuses radially from the well, a precipitin ring or 'halo' is formed at the distance where optimal proportions of antigen and antibody are achieved. The concentration of antigen is directly related to the square of the ring diameter. Unknown samples are determined by reference to a calibration curve constructed using three reference antigen standards. This method is convenient for small numbers of samples, is comparatively sensitive and reliable, although results are not usually read before 48 hours.

9.7.2 Detection of antibodies to extrinsic antigens

Antibodies to microorganisms

Detection of antimicrobial antibodies is used in the diagnosis of infection, in the investigation of immune deficiency, and in determining the response to vaccination with microorganisms (e.g., polio virus) or their products (e.g., tetanus toxoid). With respect to bacterial infection, the main immunological techniques for antibody detection are: (1) direct or indirect (Coombs) agglutination of suspensions of bacteria; (2) precipitation of soluble antigen by antibody in agar; (3) complement fixation, using rabbit antibody-coated sheep erythrocytes as the indicator system – absence of haemolysis indicates complement fixation, due to an initial reaction of antibody in the patient's serum with the original (bacterial) antigen; (4) immunofluorescence – reaction of serum antibody with the antigen (organism) in smears is detected by a fluorescein-labelled anti-human immunoglobulin antibody using UV microscopy; and (5) RIA or ELISA – antibody in patient's serum is detected by binding of anti-human immunoglobulin labelled with either a radioisotope (most often ^{125}I) or an enzyme (e.g., horseradish peroxidase or alkaline phosphatase) which produces a colour change in the presence of the appropriate substrate (see Section 9.2.3).

A similar spectrum of assays (3–5 above) is available for serological detection of virus-specific antibodies. More sensitive assays, such as RIA and ELISA, especially those which detect virus-specific IgM, are replacing the classical complement fixation test. In addition, antibody to the many viruses which agglutinate erythrocytes can be detected by haemagglutination inhibition. Anti-viral antibodies can also be detected by neutralization of viral cytopathic effects on cultured cells (viral neutralization test).

Antibodies to non-replicating antigens

The tests used to detect and quantify antibodies to non-invasive antigens, such as grass pollen, fungal antigens or food allergens, depend on: (1) the type of immune (hypersensitivity) reaction elicited by the antigen, and (2) the class of immunoglobulin mediating the response.

In immediate (type I) hypersensitivity (see Chapter 1, Section 1.7) intradermal 'prick' tests performed on the forearm are useful in establishing that an IgE-mediated response is involved and in identifying the offending allergen(s) from an antigen panel. These tests are of value in the investigation of extrinsic asthma, hay fever, and anaphylactic reactions to various substances. Normal serum levels of IgE are extremely low and antigen-specific IgE antibodies must be quantified by a high sensitive assay—the radio-allergosorbent test (RAST). This test is identical to a standard radio-immunoassay, except that the antigen (allergen) is coated on to (covalently bound to) cellulose discs rather than a plate resulting in very high sensitivity. Test serum (IgE) is added, then unbound protein washed away, the bound antibody is detected by a radiolabelled anti-IgE.

9.8 Assessment of complement

Complement represents one of the major effector systems recruited by humoral immune reactions to deal with antigen elimination and individuals who have defects in their complement system, suffer from various disease syndromes. Tests of complement measure are: (1) the functional activity of the system using antibody-coated red blood cells as targets (i.e., the antigen-antibody complex). The activated complement proteins result in the lysis of the red cells, associated with the terminal components C8 and C9. Spectrophotometric measurement of the released haemoglobulin relates to the haemolytic capacity of complement from freshly collected blood, in a standardized assay. Thus the assay allows a numerical documentation of total functional (haemolytic) complement which is related to a normal population range. Total functional complement is low in severe immune complex disease (e.g., very active SLE); it is very low or absent in rare genetic complement deficiency disorders; (2) ELISA and RIA assays are used for detection of complement activation products; and (3) the immunochemical measurement of C3 and C4 (see Chapter 1, Section 1.5.1) and other components is made possible by the use of specific anti-sera, using simple tests, such as radial immunodiffusion or more expensive auto-analyser machines.

9.9 Recombinant DNA technology

9.9.1 Introduction

Recombinant DNA technology is a powerful tool of molecular biology and is allowing the definition of pathology at the cellular and molecular level with a hitherto undreamt of precision. It is also providing laboratory-derived 'genes' and their products for diagnosis, therapy, and disease prevention. The technology refers to the ability to isolate one form of DNA (e.g., human) and to link it to another (e.g., microbial DNA). The derived hybrid DNA can then be used to increase production of human DNA in amounts which can then be isolated (i.e., cloning of the DNA). The 'recombined' DNA complex can provide ample material for direct analyses but it can also be induced in certain *in vitro* systems to transcribe its mRNA and translate its encoded protein product. Recently, recombinant DNA has been used experimentally to introduce foreign genes into the germ line of rodent embryos to generate so called transgenic animals, facilitating the *in vivo* analyses of the functioning of the introduced gene. Such technological advances have brought to the forefront the concept of gene therapy. As DNA comprises the genes within the chromosomes the technology is also referred to as 'gene cloning' or 'genetic engineering'.

Outlined below are selected areas of some of the principles, tools, and methodologies of recombinant DNA technology together with examples of its useful exploitation in medicine and immunology.

9.9.2 The basis of recombinant DNA technology

Deoxyribonucleic acid (DNA) has a double helical structure with a backbone of sugars and phosphates, the two strands being held together by the specific pairing of the nucleotide bases, adenine (A), thymine (T), cytosine (C), and guanine (G).

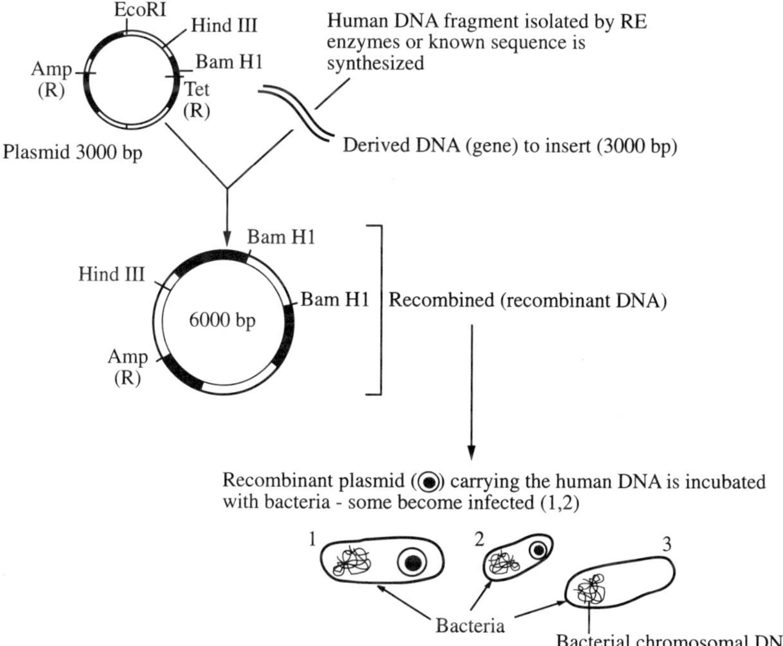

Fig. 9.7. Recombinant DNA technology: RE (restriction endonuclease) enzymes, e.g., Eco RI, Hind III, are used to cleave DNA (human and plasmid). Human DNA than ligated to plasmid DNA (6000 bp (base pairs)). Plasmid-infected bacteria (1, 2) are selected by growth in media with antibiotics (e.g., ampicillin) which favour their survival over non plasmid carrying bacteria (3).

Triple codes of bases (e.g., ATG, CCT) encode the information for single amino acids and a precise genetic code exists for the instruction to synthesize proteins as outlined below.

$$\text{DNA} \xrightarrow{\textit{Transcription}} \text{RNA} \xrightarrow{\textit{Translation}} \text{Protein}$$

Reverse flow of information was found to be possible when the *enzyme reverse transcriptase* (RT) was defined in certain retroviruses in the 1970s (see also Chapter 8):

$$\text{DNA} \xleftarrow[\substack{\uparrow \\ \text{RT}}]{} \text{RNA}$$

Mutation of DNA is either induced by external agents or may occur spontaneously. Mutation can be associated with base changes, deletions, and many other genetic mechanisms culminating in the absence of, or the presence of an aberrant/defective gene and its protein product and thus ultimately result in the expression of disease.

DNA within a cell nucleus (the genome) is extremely coiled (supercoiled) and comprises several thousands of millions of base pairs, each of the 46 chromosomes (23 pairs) themselves possess tens of millions of bases, the individual genes making up a chromosome may be comprised of tens of thousands to several millions of bases. Thus, to study systematically and to isolate genes, requires special methods of handling and fragmenting DNA in a controllable and defined manner.

Recombinant DNA technology requires:

1. Defined sources and forms of DNA and restriction enzymes.
2. Cell systems for its cloning.

9.9.3 Sources of DNA and restriction endonucleases

1. *Nuclear DNA* is extracted from cells using standard physical and biochemical methods. The large nuclear DNA can be broken into fragments using a series of bacteria-derived enzymes called restriction endonucleases (RE), the enzymes show a specificity for certain base sequences where they will 'cut' the DNA. REs have many acronyms, e.g., EcoRI, Hind III, Bam H1, defined by the bacteria from which they are isolated (Eco—from *Escherichia coli*). Such RE-derived fragments of DNA can be used to define an individual's genetic identity (DNA finger-printing) as well as to define polymorphisms in the population (i.e., variation in the cutting sequences between individuals—so-called *restriction fragment length polymorphism* (RFLPs). When the genomic location of a disease gene is not known DNA markers may be defined near to the gene which can be shown by inheritance studies to be co-inherited at all times with the gene. Thus a map of RFLPs

can be used to define the presence of a linked disease gene. RFLPs are inherited in a simple Mendelian fashion.

2. *Messenger RNA* extracted from the cytoplasm of cells can be incubated with the reverse transcriptase enzyme together with appropriate bases, sugars and added phosphates, to generate DNA by reverse pattern of synthesis.

3. *Synthetic DNA* genes can be manufactured in the laboratory in an automated manner. The method depends on knowing the base sequences of a particular gene. If a protein is known and its amino acid profile is sequenced (also possible by automation), then the triple code of the encoded DNA is deducible. The code can then be used in an automated system to manufacture the gene.

4. Small amounts of isolated DNA can be significantly increased by using the *polymerase chain reaction (PCR) technique.*

9.9.4 Plasmids: cloning DNA

Cell systems for cloning DNA

Within some bacteria is found not only chromosomal DNA but also circular (non-chromosomal) DNA which are called plasmids. Plasmids represent the simplest autonomous (replicating) life forms. Plasmids will infect bacteria, other than the ones in which they are already present, with high efficiency. On infecting the bacterial cell the plasmid will use the cell's machinery as an efficient way of replicating its DNA to high levels commensurate with the massive exponential replication growth of bacteria. Plasmids have been known to microbiologists for many years as the sources of transmission of antibiotic resistance between bacteria. For the 'genetic engineer' a plasmid can be constructed—'engineered'—to incorporate foreign DNA (e.g., human DNA). It thus becomes the ideal vector. Such is indeed the achievement exploited in recombinant technology, as shown in Fig. 9.7.

The circular form of the plasmid can be cut open with an appropriate RE as shown in Fig. 9.7. If the same enzyme is used to cut human DNA, the cut ends of both species of DNA will be matching and the human DNA can be ligated to the plasmid DNA (using a ligase enzyme). The 'recombinant' plasmid is then used to infect bacteria, which during their multiplication make many identical copies of the plasmid and its passenger human DNA. Thus, cloned human DNA (genes) is obtained. Other vectors include bacteriophages, and hybrid constructs of bacteriophages with plasmids are called cosmids.

9.9.5 Uses of cloned DNA (genes)

1. *Gene probes to analyse genetic diseases.* Many single gene defect diseases (as defined by classical Mendelian inheritance studies) have been characterized at the molecular level (e.g., haemoglobinopathies, antithrombin III deficiency, and some immune deficiency syndromes), and the defective genes cloned. Analysis of base sequences in the cloned DNA has revealed mechanisms, such as base deletions, insertions, inversions, and mutation of regulatory gene sequences, as fundamental mechanisms, in aetiopathology.

Additionally, such cloned genes can be radiolabelled and used as probes to seek and define the presence of the abnormal gene in family studies for carrier status, and in pre-natal diagnosis. Cells from various tissues are obtained from the individuals under investigation and the DNA is extracted by standard physical and biochemical techniques. It is then denatured by heating. The denatured strands can be 'cut up' by selected REs. The fragments are separated by molecular size on gel transferred to a solid support phase by a process called *Southern blotting*. The fragments are then exposed to the labelled (single strand) gene probe in renaturing conditions. DNA when exposed to temperatures significantly above normal unfolds and its strands separate—if returned to renaturing conditions the strands will reassociate but with precise restricted complementarity as defined and dictated by the matching base sequences. If the complementary sequence (the disease gene sequence) is present in the DNA preparation it will hybridize (make the double strand) with the single stranded DNA probe (also referred to as cDNA-complementary DNA). Many gene probes are now available for defining a significant number of diseases.

2. *Labelled gene probes* can be used *in vitro* to bind *in situ* to cells, or chromosome preparations (metaphase) to define unknown chromosomal location of genes. Such a strategy, using recombinant-derived cDNA for immunoglobulin and T cell receptor genes, has resulted in the definition of their respective locations. Where the chromosome has been known to be associated with a certain disease (e.g., diseases inherited and expressed in males only, thus the gene must be on the female X chromosome) recombinant DNA constructs have contributed, together with family studies of diseased individuals, in precisely defining the unknown gene and its position on the chromosome. Such a strategy has recently resulted in the successful characterization and cloning of the gene for Duchenne muscular dystrophy (DMD) (on the X chromosome). More exacting molecular genetics and technologies have also recently resulted in the cloning of the cystic fibrosis gene from chromosome 7. The ability to define such genes, apart from their

usefulness in diagnosis (pre-natal), should allow definition of the cellular defects and possible new therapies.

3. *Recombinant DNA-derived genes* have been inserted into so-called expression systems (bacteria and yeasts) whereby gene transcription and translation occurs with production of pure, encoded protein. This approach has resulted in the production of recombinant DNA-derived proteins, such as human insulin, various cytokines including IL-1 to IL-8 and the interferons α, β, and γ, erythropoietin, Factor VIII, and growth hormone, and also the enzyme streptokinase for thrombolytic therapy. Most of these cloned products are being used in human therapy (see Chapters 1 and 7). Also, novel vaccines and antibodies are being produced for clinical use by the application of recombinant DNA technology (see Chapter 1).

4. *Recombinant DNA-derived sequences* have allowed the definition of *proto-oncogenes and oncogenes* involved in the aetiology of cancer. Such cloned, active genes have been used to transform cells *in vitro* in order to study some of the aetiological mechanisms involved in carcinogenesis in fairly precise molecular terms. Thus, the pivotal role of oncogenes, such as K-ras, has been defined in bowel cancers and the C-erbB2 oncogene in breast cancer. Experimental results have indicated the oncogenes to be significant prognostic indicators.

5. *Complex diseases* involving the interaction of genetic and environmental factors, e.g., MHC-associated diseases and cardiovascular disease, have been partially defined aetiologically at the molecular level by the use of recombinant DNA analysis. Thus, MHC association in diseases such as type I insulin-dependent diabetes have become precisely characterized with respect to inherited DNA sequences defineable with extracted DNA from patients. Defective or aberrant genes encoding the lipoproteins and their receptors have been recently associated with the development of certain forms of cardiovascular disease, including the tendency for aortic aneurysm formation.

6. As mentioned, recent experiments have been performed whereby cloned genes have been introduced into the germ line (into sex cells—therefore inheritable for generations) of experimental animals. Such *transgenic animals* have established that deficiencies such as growth hormone can be amenable to gene therapy. The problems (ethical, biotechnological) surrounding the possibility of such approaches in human are complex and immense. As revealed by the animal experiments we know very little of the complex *in vivo* regulatory mechanisms involved in gene control and expression in different cells. Good therapy will require much more than just insertion and expresson of cloned genes; they will have to be carefully

regulated, medically and ethically. Many authorities doubt that germ line gene therapy is feasible or acceptable in humans. Contrastingly, *somatic gene therapy*—whereby a targeted defective cell is manipulated to have a gene inserted to correct a defined gene defect within that cell and that individual (i.e., it is not inherited in the offspring)—is seen as more acceptable to alleviate human suffering and disease. Immune deficiency diseases involving certain defined gene defects in T and B cells are seen as good targets for somatic gene therapy. Thus, the defective gene can be replaced by direct insertion of the normal gene into bone marrow cells, particularly the lymphoid stem cell, hence replacing the defect and permitting normal T and B lymphocyte development and function. Methods for directly inserting genes into cells (so-called transfection techniques) use various physico-chemical approaches, including micro-injection, use of Ca^{2+} salts, and modified viral constructs—all with variable degrees of efficiency and predictability.

Significant methodological problems, as well as ethical, personal, and international considerations will need to be addressed and defined before gene therapy becomes established in clinical practice—but established it will be.

References and Further reading

Chapel, H. and Gooi, H.C. (1990). *Clinical immunology—a practical approach.* (1st edn). Oxford University Press. Oxford.

Polak, J.M. and Von Noorden, S. (ed.) (1986). *Immunocytochemistry—modern methods and applications* (2nd edn). Wright, London.

Glossary

Acquired tolerance Immunological phenomenon consisting of the inability (acquired) of an individual to respond to a particular antigen.

Activation marker Molecule expressed on the cell surface indicating activation of the cell (e.g., interleukin-2 receptor).

Acute phase response Enhanced rates of synthesis of certain serum proteins (e.g., C-reactive protein (CRP) and most of the complement components) during inflammation which rapidly protect the host against microorganisms. The acute phase response is induced by agents such as IL-1, IL-6, and TNF, and is an important non-specific defence mechanism.

ADCC (antibody-dependent cellular cytotoxicity) A cytotoxic reaction in which Fc receptor-bearing killer cells recognize target cells coated with specific antibodies. Cells that mediate ADCC have been called killer (*K*) cells and are composed of a heterogeneous group of cells.

Adhesion molecule *See*, e.g., intercellular adhension molecule-1 (I-CAM1).

Adjuvant Substance that enhances, non-specifically, the immune response to an antigen. An adjuvant is usually administered with antigen, but may also be given before or after antigen. *See*, e.g., Freund's adjuvant.

Affinity A measure of the binding strength between two molecules (e.g., an antigenic determinant and an antibody-combining site).

AIDS (acquired immunodeficiency syndrome) Form of immunodeficiency resulting from infection with a lymphocytotropic virus (human immunodeficiency virus—HIV). HIV infection can cause profound lymphopenia, primarily of $CD4^{+}$ T lymphocytes. Affected individuals are extremely susceptible to opportunistic infections and may acquire certain malignancies.

Agglutination Clumping of particulate antigens (e.g., red blood cells, bacteria) by antibodies. Agglutination may be observed grossly or microscopically, and may be used as a test to detect the presence of and/or measure the level of antigen or antibody.

Allele Alternative form of a gene at a particular genetic locus.

Allelic exclusion Expression in a single cell, of only one allele at a particular locus. Allelic exclusion is characteristic of the expression of immunoglobulin genes.

Allergen Antigen that induces allergy. Common environmental allergens are globular proteins in pollens, animal danders, insect venoms, and various foods.

Allergy Altered immune reactivity to commonly encountered environmental antigens.

Alloantigen Antigen found only in some members of a species, e.g., blood group substances, HLA antigens.

Allogeneic Referring to genetic variants within a species.

Allograft Graft to a genetically different member of the same species. Allografts are rejected mainly by virtue of an immunological response of T lymphocytes to histocompatibility antigens.

Allotype The protein product of an allele that may be detected as an antigen by another member of the same species.

Alternative pathway of complement One of two possible mechanisms (the other being the classical pathway) for the activation of C3.

ANAS (anti-nuclear antibodies) Antibody to DNA, RNA, histone or non-histone proteins found in the serum of individuals, particularly those with certain auto-immune diseases.

Anaphylatoxin Complement peptides (C3a and C5a) which cause mast cell degranulation and smooth muscle contraction.

Anaphylaxis An antigen-specific immune reaction mediated primarily by IgE, which results in vasodilation and constriction of smooth muscles, including those of the bronchus, and which may result, in extreme cases, in the death of the individual.

Anergy Absence of an expected immune response. This term is used in clinical medicine to describe the diminished delayed type hypersensitivity (DTH) found in some disease states. Anergy is usually demonstrated by skin tests with ubiquitous antigens.

Antibody (AB) Protein that is produced in response to stimulation by antigen and that reacts specifically with that antigen.

Antigen (Ag) A molecule which reacts with antibody.

Antigen presentation The process by which certain cells (e.g., macrophages) express antigens on their cell surfaces in a form recognizable by lymphocytes.

Antigenic determinant Portion of an antigen that makes contact with a particular antibody or T cell receptor. Most proteins probably have many determinants but, because of steric interference, only a limited number of antibodies can bind to the antigen at any one time.

Anti-idiotypic antibodies Antibodies which react with the antigenic determinants (idiotypes) on the V (variable) region of other antibodies. Because anti-idiotypes can bind to antigen receptors on T and B cells they can, in some situations, be as efficient as antigens in stimulating these cells.

APCs (antigen-presenting cells) A variety of cell types which carry antigen in a form that can stimulate lymphocytes.

'Arthus' reaction Antibody-mediated hypersensitivity reaction characterized by oedematous, haemorrhagic lesions of the skin. Occurs upon introduction of antigen into an individual with pre-existing circulating IgG antibodies. The 'arthus' reaction is an experimental model of immune complex disease (type III hypersensitivity).

Atopy The clinical manifestation of Type 1 hypersensitivity reactions, including eczema, asthma, and rhinitis, due to IgE antibodies. Approximately 10 per cent of the population manifest some form of atopy.

Autoantibody Antibody that reacts with an antigen that is a normal constituent of the tissues of the individual forming the antibody.

Autoantigen Normal constituent of the tissues of an individual that induces and reacts with an autoantibody.

Autoimmunity Condition whereby antibodies or T lymphocytes are reactive with antigenic determinants of self.

Autologous Part of the same individual. The term is used to describe self antigens or grafts taken from and returned to the same individual.

Autosome Chromosome other than the X or Y sex chromosomes.

Azathioprine Derivative of mercaptopurine, widely used in the treatment of malignant disease and for immunosuppression.

AZT (azidothymidine) *See* zidovudine.

B lymphocyte Lymphocyte that produces immunoglobulin. B cells constitute about half of all lymphocytes. In lymph nodes, B lymphocytes are localized mainly in the follicles, whereas T lymphocytes are found in the paracortex. Distinguished from T cells by the presence of membrane immunoglobulin, complement receptor 2 and by class II histocompatability molecules (not found on resting T cells).

β (β_2m-microglobulin) A monomorphic polypeptide which constitutes part of some membrane proteins, and is non-covalently linked with the MHC class I molecular complex.

BCG (bacille Calmette-Guérin) An attenuated strain of bovine *Mycobacterium tuberculosis*, used as a vaccine to protect against tuberculosis (and leprosy). It is named after the two French workers who first cultivated the organism.

Bence-Jones protein Protein in urine of patients with multiple myeloma that precipitates when heated to 45–60 °C and re-dissolves on further heating. It is the light chain of the myeloma protein found in the serum of the same patient.

Bursa of Fabricius A lymphoepithelial organ found at the junction of the hind gut and cloaca in birds which is the site of B cell maturation.

C1–C9 Components of the complement pathway which are responsible for mediating inflammatory reactions, opsonization of particles, and cell lysis.

C1q Sub-component of the C1 complex that binds to immunoglobulin and thereby initiates complement activation by the classical pathway.

C1r One of two serine esterases that are part of the C1 complex, the other being C1s.

C3a and C5a Small peptides split from the parent molecules during complement activation which act directly on phagocytes (especially neutrophils) to stimulate the respiratory burst. Both are capable of triggering mediator release from mast cells and basophils. Both (especially C5a) have chemotactic properties and increase vascular permeability.

C4 Fourth component of complement which reacts in sequence following fixation of C1 to antigen-antibody complexes.

CEA (carcino-embryonic antigen) Glycoprotein antigen on the membrane of epithelial cells of the gastrointestinal tract and structures derived from the primitive gut. CEA is present in large amounts on colo-rectal carcinoma cells and in lesser amounts on normal fetal colon cells.

CD (cluster of differentiation) Antigenic determinants on cell surface molecules of leucocytes and platelets that are detected by monoclonal antibodies.

CDR (complementarity-determining region) Segment of a variable region containing amino acid residues that determine antigen-binding specificity. Residues in CDRs often make contact with antigen.

Chemiluminescence Generation of light by a chemical reaction used in the study of phagocytosis. Light is emitted from oxidants generated in neutrophils and monocytes during the respiratory burst that occurs with phagocytosis.

Chemotaxis Reorientation and directional migration of cells in response to concentration gradients of certain chemical stimuli.

Chimerism The coexistence of cells from genetically different individuals in one body.

Class I, II, and III antigens The three major classes of molecules coded within the major histocompatibility complex (MHC). Class I molecules have one MHC-encoded peptide associated with B_2-microglobulin. Class II molecules have two MHC-encoded peptides which are non-covalently associated; Class III molecules include complement components.

Clonal selection The fundamental basis of lymphocyte activation in which antigen selectively stimulates only those cells which express receptors for it to divide and differentiate.

Clone A family of cells or organisms having a genetically identical constitution, i.e., cells derived from a single individual by asexual multiplication.

CMI (cell-mediated immunity) Immunological reactions initiated by T lymphocytes and mediated by effector T lymphocytes and macrophages.

Complement A group of serum proteins involved in the control of inflammation, the activation of phagocytes, and the lytic attack on cell membranes. The system can be activated by interaction with the immune system (classical pathway) or by the alternative pathway.

Constant regions (C domains) The relatively invariant parts of immunoglobulin heavy and light chains and the α, β, γ, and δ chains of the T cell receptor.

Coombs (antiglobulin) test Method for detecting the deposition of IgG antibodies or complement on red blood cells or for detecting the presence of circulating IgG antibodies reactive against red blood cells.

CRP (C-reactive protein) Part of the acute phase proteins, synthesized in the liver and released into the circulation, as the result of trauma/inflammation.

Cryoglobulin Immunoglobulin that precipitates when it is cooled below 37°C. Cryoglobulins are not found in normal serum but occur in certain diseases.

CSFs (colony-stimulating factors) A group of cytokines which control the differentiation of haematopoietic stem cells.

CTL (cytotoxic T lymphocyte) T lymphocyte that kills other cells.

Cyclosporin A A fungal metabolite (cyclic peptide) which selectively inhibits early events in $CD4^+$ T cell activation and lymphokine production.

Cytokines A generic term for soluble molecules which mediate interactions between cells.

Cytolysis Killing of target cells by damage to their surface membranes and release of their intracellular contents.

Cytophilic Having a propensity to bind to cells.

Cytoskeleton Network of different types of protein filaments present in the cytoplasm of eukaryotic cells. They serve as a scaffold or framework for other cell constituents and are essential for maintaining shape, internal organization, and motility of the cell.

Cytostatic Having the ability to stop cell growth and proliferation.

Cytotoxic Having the ability to kill cells.

Degranulation Exocytosis of granules from cells such as mast cells and basophils.

Dendritic cells Antigen-presenting cells in lymph nodes, spleen and (at low levels) in blood.

DTH (delayed type hypersensitivity) This term includes the delayed skin reactions associated with type IV (cell-mediated) hypersensitivity.

EBV (Epstein–Barr virus) Causal agent of Burkitt's lymphoma and infectious mononucleosis, and which has the ability to transform human B cells into stable cell lines.

Effector cells A functional concept which, in context, means those lymphocytes or phagocytes which produce the end effect.

ELISA (enzyme-linked immunosorbent assay) Method for detecting antigens or antibodies utilizing solid phase enzyme-substrate reactions.

Endocytosis Uptake by cells of materials from the extracellular fluid by means of vesicles formed from the plasma membrane. There are two types of endocytosis: receptor mediated and fluid phase endocytosis (pinocytosis).

Endosomes Intracellular vesicles formed in the process of endocytosis.

Endotoxin Synonym for heat stable lipopolysaccharides, associated with the outer membranes of Gram-negative bacteria.

Epitope A single antigenic determinant. In functional terms, it is the portion of an antigen which combines with the antibody paratope.

Exocytosis Process whereby the contents of intracellular vesicles are released into the external environment.

Exon Segment of an interrupted gene or primary RNA transcript that is represented in mature RNA.

Fab fragment The part of an antibody molecule which contains the antigen-combining site, consisting of a light chain and part of a heavy chain.

Factor B Heat-labile protein of the alternative pathway of complement, which binds to C3b.

Factor D Serine protease of the alternative pathway of complement which cleaves Factor B.

FACS (fluorescence activated cell sorter) Machine which rapidly analyses the size and fluorescence intensity of single cells stained with specific, fluorescent antibodies. The cells can then be sorted using these parameters.

Fc The portion of an antibody that is responsible for binding to antibody receptors on cells and the C1q component of complement.

Fc receptor Receptor for the Fc portion of immunoglobulin.

FK-506 An immunosuppressive fungal metabolite (macrolide antibiotic) with a similar mode of action to Cyclosporin A but more potent than the former.

Follicle Structure in lymphoid tissues characterized by loosely packed lymphocytes and antigen-presenting cells. Follicles are found in the superficial cortex of lymph nodes and the splenic white pulp, and contain mainly B cells. Unstimulated lymph nodes contain primary follicles, which develop into expanded, secondary follicles after antigen stimulation.

Follicular dendritic cells Cells located in the follicles of lymph node and spleen characterized by the presence of many thin cytoplasmic extensions between closely packed B lymphocytes.

Freund's adjuvant An emulsion of aqueous antigen in oil. Freund's complete adjuvant (FCA) also contains killed *Mycobacterium* tuberculosis, which Freund's incomplete adjuvant does not.

Genotype Genetic constitution in an organism; not all of it is expressed in the individual.

Germinal centre Regions of rapidly proliferating cells seen in the centre of some secondary lymphoid follicles.

Graft versus host disease Condition caused by allogeneic donor lymphocytes reaction against host tissue in an immunologically compromised recipient.

Granulocyte White blood cell of myeloid lineage, characterised by a nucleus composed of distinct lobes that are connected by thin strands of chromatin. Also called polymorphonuclear leucocyte (PMNL).

Graves' disease Autoimmune disease that results in hyperthyroidism. Patients may have an IgG autoantibody (known as long-acting thyroid stimulator, LATS) to the thyroid-stimulating hormone (TSH) receptor.

Haplotype A set of genetic determinants located on a single chromosome.

Hapten A small molecule which can act as an epitope but is incapable, by itself, of eliciting an antibody response.

Heavy chain Larger polypeptide chain in an immunoglobulin molecule.

Heterodimer Protein composed of two different chains.

Histocompatibility The ability of an individual to accept grafts from another individual.

HIV (human immunodeficiency virus) Retrovirus that causes AIDS and related disorders. The virus infects mainly T lymphocytes of the $CD4^+$ subset in which the virus can be latent or lytic. HIV also infects $CD4^+$ mononuclear phagocytes.

HLA (human leucocyte antigen) The human major histocompatibility complex encoded and expressed molecules.

Humoral Pertaining to the extracellular fluids including the serum and lymph.

Hybridoma Cell line created *in vitro* by fusion of two different cells, one a lymphocyte, and the other a tumour cell (myeloma).

Hypersensitivity An immune response to a previously encountered antigen which occurs in an exaggerated or inappropriate form—four types described.

Type I (immediate) hypersensitivity is manifested within minutes of exposure to antigen and is dependent on the binding of antigen to IgE on the surface of mast cells and the degranulation of these cells (e.g., allergic asthma, hay fever).

Type II (antibody-mediated) hypersensitivity is caused by antibody reacting with cell surface antigens which sensitizes the cells for antibody-dependent cell-mediated cytotoxicity (ADCC) by killer (K) cells or lysis by complement (e.g., destruction of red blood cells in transfusion reactions).

Type III (immune complex-mediated) hypersensitivity is due to the deposition of antigen-antibody complexes in tissues and blood vessels, the activation of complement with consequent attraction of polymorphs resulting in tissue damage (e.g., extrinsic allergic alveolitis).

Type IV (delayed or cell-mediated) hypersensitivity is mediated by antigen-sensitized T cells which, following contact with antigen, release lymphokines. These attract and activate macrophages, causing tissue damage.

Hypervariable regions The most variable areas (in amino acid sequences) of the V domains of immunoglobulin and T cell receptor chains. These regions are clustered at the distal portion of the V domain and contribute to the antigen-binding site.

Ia antigen Class II histocompatibility molecule, initially defined as 'I region-associated' antigen.

I-CAM1 (intercellular adhesion molecule 1) Cell surface glycoprotein found on endothelial, dendritic and many other cell types and which is the ligand for lymphocyte function-associated antigen-1 (LFA-1) which is present on T cells.

Idiotope A single antigenic determinant on an antibody V region.

Idiotype The antigenic characteristic of the V region of an antibody.

IFNs (interferons) A group of mediators which increase the resistance of cells to viral infection, and act as cytokines. There are three types: IFN-α and IFN-β, produced by leucocytes and fibroblasts; and IFN-γ, produced by activated T cells. IFN also modulates immune responses and enhances natural killer (NK) cell activity.

Immune complex The product of an antigen-antibody reaction which may also contain complement components.

Immune response (Ir) genes Genes that control the immune response of T lymphocytes to proteins and synthetic polypeptides.

Immune surveillance Concept that the immune system eliminates cells that express aberrant or neoantigens as a result of somatic mutation or the action of carcinogens.

Immuno-electrophoresis Technique combining electrophoresis and immunodiffusion. It is usually carried out in a gel medium, such as agar. Thus, antigens are characterized by both electrophoretic mobility and antigenic properties. The technique is very effective in identifying components in complex mixtures.

Immunofixation Technique for detecting specific antigens in a complex mixture of proteins that have been separated by electrophoresis. After electrophoresis, the gel is flooded with antibodies, washed to remove soluble antigens and antibodies, and then stained to detect antigen-antibody precipitates.

Immunofluorescence Technique used to identify particular antigen microscopically in tissues or on cells by the binding of a fluorescent antibody conjugate.

Immunoglobulin Protein that has antibody activity.

Integrins Glycoproteins on the cell membrane that act as receptors for extracellular matrix glycoproteins, blood proteins, and other cell surface glycoproteins. Integrins serve, in general, as transmembrane links between extracellular ligands and cytoskeleton. They are presumed to facilitate cell migration in embryos, wound healing, phagocytosis, and target cell killing.

Interdigitating dendritic cells These are located in the T cell area of lymph nodes, and carry MHC class II molecules and are highly active in presenting antigen to T helper cells. They are thought to be most important in the development of contact (delayed) hypersensitivity reactions.

Interleukins (IL-1–IL-10) A group of molecules (cytokines) secreted mainly by mononuclear cells and involved in signalling between cells of the immune system.

Interleukins induce growth and differentiation of lymphocytes and pluripotential haematopoietic stem cells.

Introns Gene segments which lie between the exons. They do not encode protein but contain sequences important in gene control and the process of recombination.

Isotype Refers to genetic variation within a family of proteins or peptides such that every member of the species will have each isotype of the family represented in its genome (e.g., immunoglobulin classes).

J chain Monomorphic polypeptide present in and required for the polymerization of polymeric IgA and IgM.

K (killer) cells A group of cells which are able to destroy their targets by antibody-dependent cell-mediated cytotoxicity and which bear Fc receptors.

K562 Cell line from a patient with chronic myelogenous leukaemia, commonly used as targets in *in vitro* assays of natural killer (NK) cell activity.

LAK (lymphokine-activated killer) cells Cytotoxic lymphocytes with a wide repertoire of cellular targets, generated by interaction with IL-2.

Langerhans cells Antigen-presenting cells of the skin which emigrate to local lymph nodes to become dendritic cells; they are very active in presenting antigen to T cells. They have a characteristic racket-shaped granule called the Birbeck granule (function unknown), and are rich in MHC class II molecules.

LATS (long-acting thyroid stimulator) *See* Graves' disease.

Leukotrienes A collection of metabolites of arachidonic acid produced by the lipo-oxygenase pathway, generating mediators of acute inflammation and the slow reacting substances important in hypersensitivity.

LFAs (leucocyte functional antigens) A group of three molecules (LFA1–3) which mediate intercellular adhesion between leucocytes and other cells in a non-specific manner.

LGLs (large granular lymphocytes) A group of morphologically defined (azurophilic granules) lymphocytes, containing the majority of killer (K) cell and natural killer (NK) cell activity.

Light chain Small polypeptide chain in a heterodimer. As used by immunologists, the term usually refers to the light chain of an immunoglobulin molecule.

Loci The positions on a chromosome at which a particular gene is found.

LPS (lipopolysaccharide) A polyclonal B cell mitogen in mice which induces immunoglobulin secretion. It is derived from the cell wall of Gram-negative bacteria.

Lymphoblast Large cell of lymphocyte lineage that contains a nucleolus and synthesizes DNA.

Lymphoid Referring to lymphocytes or to tissues that contain large accumulations of lymphocytes.

Lymphokine A generic term for molecules other than antibodies which are involved in signalling between cells of the immune system and are produced by lymphocytes.

Lysosomes Enzyme containing organelles present in cells, in macrophages important in the breakdown and digestion of phagocytosed material.

Lysozyme (muramidase) An enzyme which digests a bond in the cell wall proteoglycan of some Gram-positive bacteria.

MABs (monoclonal antibodies) Antibodies produced by a single clone and which are homogeneous.

Mantoux test Test for cell-mediated immunity to tuberculosis in which tuberculin is injected intradermally.

MDP (muramyl dipeptide) The smallest adjuvant active part of the BCG (bacillus Calmette-Guérin) extractable from the cell wall.

MHC (major histocompatibility complex) A genetic region found in all mammals whose products are primarily responsible for functional signalling between lymphocytes and cells expressing antigen. MHC molecules are also involved in the rejection of grafts between individuals.

Microglial cells Itinerant phagocytes of the brain.

Mitogens Molecules which induce polyclonal differentiation and division (mitosis) of cells. A few are commonly used to induce lymphocyte subset activation and transformation, e.g., LPS, PHA, CON A, PWM.

MLR (mixed lymphocyte reaction) A technique for typing or measuring the interaction between cells *in vitro*, in which lymphocytes from different individuals are co-cultured. If the cells differ they are stimulated to undergo blast transformation and to divide. The T lymphocytes react against the MHC class I determinants on the surface of the other population.

Myeloma Plasma cell tumour produced from cells of the B cell lineage, which secretes immunoglobulin, of limited clonality.

Neoantigen Newly expressed antigenic determinant. For example, as a result of conformational change in a protein, cell transformation, complex formation of two or more molecules, or cleavage of a molecule.

NK (natural killer) cells A group of lymphocytes (predominantly Fc receptor-bearing LGL) which have the intrinsic ability to recognize and destroy some virally infected cells and various tumour cells to which the individual has not previously been sensitized.

Oncofetal antigens Antigens normally expressed in fetal life which reappear in tumours and may be secreted into the circulation.

Oncogene Gene that brings about or contributes to the neoplastic transformation of cells, e.g., c-*erb*, K-*ras*, c-*myc*.

Opportunistic infection Infections that occur mainly in patients with defects in cell-mediated immunity.

Opsonins Molecules which bind both to particles to be phagocytosed and to receptors on phagocytic cells, so acting as a bridge between the two, e.g., IgG, C3b, and CRP.

Opsonization This occurs when particles, microoganisms, or immune complexes become coated with molecules which make them more easily phagocytosed, i.e., coated with opsonins.

Peyer's patches Collections of lymphocytes in the wall of the small intestine which appear macroscopically as pale patches on the gut wall. They contain B and T cell areas and may have germinal centres.

Phagocytosis The process by which cells engulf material and enclose it within a vacuole (phagosome) in the cytoplasm.

Phenotype The expressed characteristics of an individual, i.e., depends on the genotype and how the genes are expressed.

Plasma cell An antibody-producing B lymphocyte which has reached the end of its differentiation pathway.

Polyclonal activator Substance that stimulates T or B lymphocytes, regardless of their antigen specificity.

Polyclonal antibodies Antibodies derived from many different clones of antibody-forming cells, all of which react with a particular antigen. Immunization usually results in a polyclonal antibody response.

Polymorphonuclear granulocyte Cells recognizable by their multi-lobed nuclei and numerous cytoplasmic granules. They constitute the majority of blood leucocytes.

Properdin Protein of the alternative complement pathway. It binds to the alternative pathway C3 convertase (C3bBb) and stabilizes it.

RAST (radio-allergosorbent test) A specialized form of RIA for detecting antigen-specific IgE, in which antigen is convalently coupled to cellulose discs. Antigen-specific IgE binding to the disc is detected using radiolabelled anti-IgE.

Rebuck skin window Technique for observing the evolution of inflammation. Skin is injured by scraping and coverslips are successively applied to the abrasion. These are then removed and stained to determine the types of cells present at the site of injury.

Recall antigens Antigens of common microbial pathogens are used in skin testing for delayed hypersensitivity (e.g., *Candida albicans*, PPD, streptokinase-streptodornase, mumps antigens).

Recombinant proteins The product of the process by which genetic information is rearranged during meiosis, called recombination. This process also occurs during the somatic rearrangements of DNA which occur in the formation of genes encoding antibody molecules and T cell antigen receptors. The term is also used to describe the genetically engineered proteins generated *in vitro* using isolated DNA and various expression systems.

Reticuloendothelial cells Long-lived phagocytic cells distributed throughout the organs of the body. They are derived from bone marrow stem cells and most have been shown to have receptors for the Fc region of immunoglobulin and activated C3. Their function is to scavenge antigenic particles and debris. Some of them have the ability to present antigen to lymphocytes.

(RF) Rheumatoid factor Autoantibody to IgG or IgA, usually of the IgM class, found most frequently in serum of patients with rheumatoid arthritis.

RFLP (restriction fragment length polymorphism) Polymorphism in the genome that is detected by comparing restriction maps of DNAs from different individuals. Variations in position of restriction sites (i.e., sites where restriction endonucleases cleave the DNA) may be detected as differences in lengths of restriction fragments, as revealed by Southern blotting with suitable molecular hybridization probes.

RIA (radio-immunoassay) Includes a variety of techniques which use radiolabelled reagents to detect antigen or antibody. Antibody may be detected using plates sensitized with antigen. Test antibody is applied and this is detected by the addition of a radiolabelled ligand specific for that antibody. The amount of ligand bound to the plate is proportional to the amount of test antibody.

Serotype Antigenic variant within a bacterial species identified using antibodies to surface antigenic determinants of the variants.

Somatic mutation A process occurring during B cell maturation and affecting the antibody gene region, which permits refinement of antibody specificity.

Southern blotting Technique for detecting particular sequences in a mixture of DNA fragments, usually obtained by digestion with one or more restriction endonucleases, that have been separated, according to size by gel electrophoresis. The resulting fragments are denatured and 'blotted' on to a sheet of nitrocellulose or nylon filter that is laid on top of the gel. The DNA in the filter is then hybridized with an appropriate labelled probe which hybridizes to complementary sequences in the fragements. Unbound probe is washed away, and the location of the hybridized probe is revealed by autoradiography.

Stem cells Primitive pluripotent, haematopoetic cells within the bone marrow and yolk sac.

Suppressor cells A sub-population of cells believed to be mainly T cells which act to reduce the immune responses of other T cells or B cells. Suppression may be antigen-specific, idiotype-specific, or non-specific in different circumstances.

Syngeneic Strains of animals produced by repeated inbreeding so that each pair of autosomes within an individual is identical.

TCR (T cell antigen receptor complex) Protein on the surface of T cells that specifically recognizes molecules of the MHC, either alone or in association with foreign antigens. In the cell membrane, the TCR is composed of the antigen-specific T cell receptor molecule (Ti) and is closely associated with the CD3 complex, which is believed to mediate signal transduction when the T cell receptor is engaged. Ti consists of two distinct, membrane-embedded polypeptide heterodimer chains, either α/β or γ/δ.

T lymphocyte Cell that matures in the thymus and is responsible for cell-mediated immunity and the regulation of growth and differentiation of other immunocompetent cells (e.g., B cells, mononuclear phagocytes). Mature T cells can be divided into two major subsets that differ broadly in function on the basis of surface antigenic determinants: (1)-CD4 (mainly helper-inducer T cells); and (2) CD8 (mainly cytotoxic and/or suppressor cells.)

TNF (tumour necrosis factor) Cytokine released by activated macrophages which induces leucocytosis, fever, weight loss, the acute phase reaction, and necrosis of some tumours. TNF-α (cachectin) and TNF-β (lymphotoxin) are homologous proteins, having approximately 30 per cent amino acid identity; they bind to the same receptor and share biological activities.

Tolerance A state of specific immunological unresponsiveness.

Transgenic organism Organism carrying and usually expressing an exogenous gene in its genome. In mice, the gene is usually introduced by micro-injection of a recently fertilized egg.

Transformation Morphological changes in a lymphocyte associated with the onset of division (blast transformation). Also denotes the conversion of cells in culture to a state of unrestrained growth (malignant transformation).

V domains The *N*-terminal domains of antibody heavy and light chains and the α, β, γ, and δ chains of the T cell receptor which vary between different clones and form the antigen-binding site.

VLA (very late appearing antigens) Five distinct heterodimers of cell membranes that share a common chain but have different β chains. They may function as cell matrix adhesion receptors (e.g., VLA-5 is the fibronectin receptor).

Xenogeneic Referring to interspecies antigenic differences.

Xenograft Graft to a member of a different species. Xenografts are usually rejected within a few days by antibodies and cytotoxic T lymphocytes to histocompatibility antigens.

Zidovudine (3-azido-3-deoxythymidine, – AZT) Analogue of thymidine that inhibits reverse transcriptase. It is being used in the treatment of AIDS and HIV infection.

Abbreviations

Ab	antibody
ADCC	antibody-dependent cellular cytotoxicity
AIDS	acquired immunodeficiency syndrome
Ag	antigen
ALG	anti-lymphocyte globulin
ANA	anti-nuclear antibody
APC	antigen-presenting cell
ARDS	adult respiratory distress syndrome
AS	ankylosing spondylitis
AZT	azidothymidine
BCG	Bacille Calmette Guérin
B_2M	B_2 microglobulin
CALLA	common acute lymphoblastic leukaemia antigen
CEA	carcino-embryonic antigen
CD	clusters of differentiation
CDR	complementarity-determining region
CMI	cell-mediated immunity
CML	cell-mediated lympholysis
CON A	concanavalin A
CRP	C-reactive protein
CSF	colony-stimulating factor
CTL	cytotoxic lymphocyte
CsA	Cyclosporin A
DTH	delayed type hypersensitivity
EFA	essential fatty acid
ELISA	enzyme-linked immunoabsorbent assay
EBV	Epstein–Barr virus
FACS	fluorescence activated cell sorter
FCA	Freund's complete adjuvant
FDC	follicular dendritic cell
GPC	gastric parietal cell

GVHD	graft versus host disease
HDL	high density lipoprotein
HIV	human immunodeficiency virus
HLA	human leucocyte antigen
IDDM	insulin-dependent diabetes mellitus
IFA	instrinsic factor
IFN	interferon
Ig	immunoglobulin
IL	interleukin
IR	immune response
ISCOM	immunostimulating complex
K	killer (cell)
LAK	lymphokine-activated killer (cell)
LATS	long-acting thyroid stimulator
LCA	leucocyte common antigen
LFA	lymphocyte functioning antigen
LGL	large granular lymphocyte
LPS	lipopolysaccharide
MAB	monoclonal antibody
MAF	macrophage-activating factor
MDP	muramyl dipeptide
MHC	major histocompatibility complex
MLC	mixed lymphocyte culture
MLR	mixed lymphocyte reaction
MLTC	mixed lymphocyte tumour culture
MOF	multiple organ failure
MPS	mononuclear phagocyte series
NK	natural killer (cell)
OSA	organ specific autoimmunity
PCV	post-capillary venule
PEM	protein energy malnutrition
PHA	phytohaemagglutinin
PG	prostaglandin
PMNL	polymorphonuclear leucocyte
PPD	purified protein derivature

PUFA	polyunsaturated fatty acid
PWM	pokeweed mitogen
RA	rheumatoid arthritis
RAST	radio-allergosorbent test
RIA	radio-immunoassay
RF	rheumatoid factor
RFLP	restriction fragment length polymorphism
RDT	recombinant DNA technology
SLE	systemic lupus erythematosus
SmIg	surface membrane immunoglobulin
TAA	tumour-associated antigen
TCR	T cell antigen receptor complex
TSA	tumour-specific antigen
TI	thymus-independent
TIL	tumour-infiltrating lymphocyte
TIM	tumour-infiltrating macrophage
TNF	tumour necrosis factor
TSA	tumour-specific antigen
TSH	thyroid stimulating hormone
TSI	thyroid-stimulating immunoglobulin
VLA	very late appearing antigens
VLDL	very low density lipoprotein

Index